SNEEZING AFTER SEX PREVENTS PREGNANCY

SNEEZING AFTER SEX PREVENTS PREGNANCY

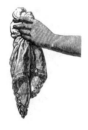

Peter Engel

ST. MARTIN'S PRESS
NEW YORK

A THOMAS DUNNE BOOK.
An imprint of St. Martin's Press.

Production Editor: David Stanford Burr

Library of Congress Cataloging-in-Publication Data

Engel, Peter H.
      Sneezing after sex prevents pregnancy / by Peter Engel.
          p.   cm.
      ISBN 0-312-14696-5
      1. Folklore—United States.   2. American wit and humor.
   3. United States—Social life and customs.   I. Title.
   GR105.E55   1996
   398'.0973—dc20   96-27926
                                                                          CIP

First Edition: December 1996

10   9   8   7   6   5   4   3   2   1

TABLE OF CONTENTS

Acknowledgments ix

A Medical Disclaimer xi

Introduction xiii

1. Time Heals All Wounds 1

2. If You Touch the Milk in Dandelions You'll
   Wet the Bed 2

3. A Spiderweb over a Crib Helps Keep a Baby Safe 3

4. Chicken Soup Cures Colds 4

5. Water Boils Faster when You Add Salt 5

6. Shock Can Turn Your Hair White Overnight 7

7. Microwave Ovens Can Make Men Sterile 8

8. A "Hair of the Dog" Will Help a Hangover 10

9. Don't Swallow Chewing Gum Because It'll
   Never Digest 11

10. Tilt Your Head Back to Stop a Nosebleed 13

11. Oatmeal Baths Are Best for Poison Ivy 14

12. Wearing Copper Jewelry Is Good for Arthritis 16

13. Using Antiperspirant Can Lead to Alzheimer's
    Disease 17

14. Rub a Potato on Your Face and Hands to
    Soften the Skin 19

15. Vitamin C Prevents Colds 20

16. A Baby Born with a Caul over Its Face Has
    Special Powers 21

17. *Redheads Have Terrible Tempers* 23
18. *Breaking a Mirror Means Seven Years of Bad Luck* 25
19. *Never Light Three on a Single Match* 26
20. *Plants in the House Mean More Oxygen* 27
21. *If You Lose Ten Pounds You'll Gain It Back* 29
22. *Opening an Umbrella Indoors Will Bring Bad Luck* 30
23. *Baldness Is Hereditary* 31
24. *The Human Body Renews Itself Every Seven Years* 33
25. *Dogs Can Sense Fear* 35
26. *Spicy Foods Give You Nightmares* 36
27. *A Woman Can't Get Pregnant while Nursing* 37
28. *Brushing Your Hair at Least One Hundred
    Strokes Will Keep It Clean* 38
29. *Women Are Most Interested in the Size of a
    Man's Penis* 39
30. *Sneezing after Sex Prevents Pregnancy* 41
31. *Take Milk Baths for Good Skin* 42
32. *Underwater Birth Ensures Babies a Happy,
    More Peaceful Life* 43
33. *Riding a Horse Can Cause a Girl to Lose Her
    Virginity* 45
34. *Cats Are Psychic* 46
35. *Once You Find Roaches in Your House You Can
    Never Get Rid of Them* 48
36. *Breast Milk Is Better for Babies Than Cow's Milk* 49
37. *Lemon Juice Will Get Rid of Freckles* 51
38. *Eat Pork Only in Months with an R in Them* 52
39. *Sit-ups Will Help Get Rid of Love Handles* 53
40. *A Woman Can't Get Pregnant during Her Period* 55
41. *Breast-feeding Prevents Breast Cancer* 56

42. *Washing Your Hair in Rainwater Makes It Cleaner*   57

43. *Suntan Oil Makes You Tan Faster*   58

44. *A Drowning Man Comes up Three Times before Staying Under*   60

45. *Dreams Predict the Future*   61

46. *Hot Toddies Help Cure a Cold or Flu*   63

47. *Being Overweight Is Caused by Overeating*   64

48. *It's Bad Luck for the Groom to See the Bride before the Wedding*   65

49. *Press a Half-dollar against a Wound to Stop the Bleeding*   67

50. *Nice Guys Finish Last*   68

51. *Famous People Die in Threes*   69

52. *You Can't Tan through a Window*   70

53. *If You Urinate on the Third Rail of the Subway Tracks, You'll Be Electrocuted*   72

54. *You Can Get AIDS or Herpes in a Hot Tub*   73

55. *You Can't Photograph into the Sun*   74

56. *Setting Out Plastic Jugs Full of Water Will Stop Dogs from Soiling Your Lawn*   76

57. *Grizzly Bears Can Be Attracted by Menstruating Women*   77

58. *If You Put Your Tongue on the Handle of a Water Pump in Winter You'll Stick to It until Spring*   79

59. *Hang a Silver Spoon in Champagne to Keep It Carbonated*   80

60. *Cracking Your Knuckles Will Give You Arthritis*   82

61. *Hitting Your Wrist with a Bible Will Make Bumps Go Away*   83

62. *Cabbage Can Reduce Breast Swelling*   84
63. *You Can Break a Glass by Singing a Certain Note*   85
64. *Bats Will Fly into Your Hair and Lay Eggs in It*   87
65. *Don't Look at an Eclipse or You'll Go Blind*   89
66. *Hot Water Freezes More Quickly than Cold Water*   90
67. *Saltpeter Will Make a Man Impotent*   92
68. *The Touch of a Menstruating Woman Makes Food Spoil*   93
69. *Crocodiles Can Grab Your Shadow and Pull You into the Water*   94
70. *You Lose Most of Your Body Heat through Your Head*   95
    Afterword   97

ACKNOWLEDGMENTS

The author wishes to recognize and thank the following for their help during the writing of this book: John Rieck, Eric Bucher, Marc Moss, Dan Barnhart, Francesca Innocenti, S. L. Daniels, Sharon Bielski, Stacy Moss, Cherilyn Parsons, Kevin McCarthy, Sherilyn Beard, Robert Van de Ven, Elena Genov, Jennifer Kortepeter, Karen Grube, Tammie Yvette Wilson, and Steve Bucher.

Thanks to Howard Cohl at Affinity Communications Corp.

A MEDICAL DISCLAIMER

Many of the tales included in this book deal with health-related issues. While we tried to find the most recent and relevant research, there is no substitute for real medical advice from a real physician. This book is intended for your entertainment and not for medical advice. Please consult a doctor for any medical problem. Do not use this book as a guideline.

Old wives are fun to listen to, but they didn't go to medical school.

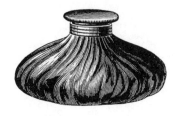

INTRODUCTION

A few years ago we published a book of old wives' tales. Its success invited a sequel.

This book is not a sequel, however, but a continuation. There are so many old wives' tales that they could not all possibly be included in any single volume of work. No matter which you include, there will always be one missing from someone's past. Admittedly (or not), we all live by certain rules and myths, if for no other reason than because they have been handed down to us. Time and retelling obscure logic and reason, but still the tales make perfect sense.

This book is not meant to discourage belief, but only to give background and explanation. If a copper ring makes your arthritis feel better, no book should dissuade you from wearing it. If you feel uncomfortable lighting three cigarettes with one match, knowing *why* may or may not change your mind. This is not our purpose. This book is meant simply to fill in some gaps in an entertaining fashion.

Why do we believe in old wives' tales? Because some are true. Many others have their roots in truth. Some are simply ridiculous and fly in the face of logic, and yet we *still* believe in them. But why? Mostly because we want to. We are convinced by the experience of others that they are true. You heard it from someone you trust, therefore it must be true. It is part of our culture, therefore it must be true.

We also have a need to put our faith in something fantastic, something unseen. Why let the reason be biology when it could be magic? It's easier to trust an old wives' tale because it will never let us down. If it fails we don't remember; when it comes true, it's notched into our memory as proof. Old wives' tales are meant to protect, not to fool, we know. They are reassuring pieces of advice from generations of women who know what's best for us.

The following pages contain some of this advice. The old wives have been around a lot longer than we have, and they still have a lot to say.

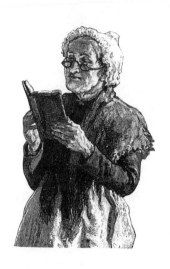

TIME HEALS ALL WOUNDS

"Time is the greatest innovator." FRANCIS BACON, *ESSAYS*, "OF INNOVATIONS"

You're in the school play and, suddenly, in front of an auditorium full of people you forget your lines. You stand frozen for what seems like an eternity and then break into tears as the audience begins to snicker. Your life is ruined, not to mention your acting career. Later that night your mother tells you, "Some day you'll look back on this and laugh."

Years later you break up with your significant other. At one point or other all your friends share the same words of wisdom with you. "All you need is a little time. You'll get over it."

The advice that time heals all wounds has its foundation in real common sense. In fact, this piece of wisdom can be traced back in writing all the way to 300 B.C. when Menander, a Greek playwright, wrote: "Time is a healer of all ills." Ben Franklin, the sage of early America, called time "an herb that cures all diseases" in his *Poor Richard's Almanac.*

What we've been told throughout history is that if enough time passes, we will gain a new and better perspective on things. Eventually you'll see that forgetting your lines in the school play was not the end of the world and that there are more fish in the sea after all.

This advice, however, assumes that the wound you have is emotional. Does it also apply to physical wounds? Well, in a way. If you get a paper cut or a black eye, then yes, over time the wound heals—with a little help from your body's own immune system and natural recuperative powers. The same can be said for the common cold, for which the only real "cure" is the time it takes for the virus to run its course.

1

Obviously this advice is meant to suggest personal perspective on a situation rather than medical guidance. Certainly there are physical and emotional conditions that time alone will not heal properly. It may take time to recover from a broken leg or an emotional trauma, but they may also need a little assistance from a physician or counselor. It's nice to know, though, that our bodies and minds do seem to heal with the help of a little time.

IF YOU TOUCH THE MILK IN DANDELIONS YOU'LL WET THE BED

"I have to pee." TOM HANKS (AS FORREST GUMP)

There you are with your loved one in a field of yellow flowers. The blanket is spread; there is a loaf of bread and a jug of wine. One of you leans back to pick a flower to present as a token of your love. After eating, you lie back and take a warm nap in the summer shade. When you wake up . . . let's just say you need a change of clothes.

Many children were warned by their overprotective parents not to let the "milk" in dandelions touch them or they'd surely wet the bed that night. Whether this superstition grew out of a hatred for a flower considered a weed or parents' frustration with chronic bed wetters, we're not sure. But, in their own way, those parents had a point.

Years ago scientists discovered that a substance found in the dandelion plant actually contains a diuretic. (A diuretic, for those unaware, helps increase the flow of urine.) Parts of the flower were boiled, made into a medicine, and used to treat patients whose urinary systems were blocked. So there actually is a connection between dandelions and urination.

Touching the flower and having it work its magic on you is another story, however. First, the amount of the diuretic you would need is more than can be found in a single flower or even an entire bouquet. And if it were enough, the diuretic has still to get into your body. It would be asking a lot for the skin to absorb that much of anything.

So pick as many dandelions for your love as you wish. You may be called a cheap date, but at least you'll be a dry one.

In the Middle Ages, the dandelion was called "pissenlit." "En lit" translates to "in bed." "Piss" translates to . . . Okay, not exactly, but it's an interesting thought, oui? Later, in sixteenth-century England, the flower was call "lion's tooth," because of its saw-tooth–edged leaves and rounded "hairy" clusters of seeds. This later became "dent-de-lion" in France, hence the name dandelion.

A SPIDERWEB OVER A CRIB HELPS KEEP A BABY SAFE

" 'Will you walk into my parlour?' said a spider to a fly:
'Tis the prettiest little parlour that ever you did spy.' "
MARY HOWITT, "THE SPIDER AND THE FLY"

You're bringing the baby home for the first time. You've got his room all ready for him. There's the crib that's been in the family for generations. The wallpaper is sky blue and has clouds and rainbows. The changing table is in place. And there, above the crib, is a spiderweb. Perfect.

You may be thinking to yourself that this may be fine childcare advice for the Addams Family, but why would anyone in their right mind want a spider's web above their sleeping baby?

This old wives' tale started back with the Chippewa Indians. They believed that a web over a crib would protect a baby while it slept by snaring any "harm" that might be nearby. The "harm" in this case was usually any evil spirits that might be flying around.

There may have been a more practical reason for having a spiderweb over a crib. Because the Chippewas made their home in the Great Lakes region, they had to live with more than evil spirits. They also had to live with mosquitos. Some researchers believe that spiderwebs may have been used as a natural mosquito net. One reason spiders make webs, after all, is to catch insects and hold them until the spider gets ready to eat. Therefore, the webs would be strong enough and durable enough to keep the insects away from the babies.

It may have been more than just a few insect bites from which the babies were protected. Mosquitos carry viruses that can cause illness, fever, and even death, especially in vulnerable infants. In that culture the symptoms of these diseases could have been seen instead as the work of evil spirits.

This is not to suggest that all new parents rush out and get a black widow for baby's room. Insect control *has* come a long way since then, and mosquitos aren't inevitable anymore. Instead, save your money for more diapers. *That* is still inevitable.

CHICKEN SOUP CURES COLDS

....

"Mmm, Mmm, good." CAMPBELL'S SOUP THEME

This guy walks out of a bar and is hit by a car. A crowd gathers around, but it's not looking good for him. Someone calls for an ambulance, but before it can arrive, from out of the crowd comes an old woman with a bowl of chicken soup. "Give him some of this," she says. The man's friend says, "Are you kidding? That won't help." "Couldn't hurt," she shrugs.

If there's anything in this world that's surely a cure for whatever ails you, it's chicken soup. From the first time we came down with a cold we were told to have a bowl. If ever there was a universally agreed upon treatment for the common cold, it's chicken soup. So it has to be true, right?

Actually, yes. We're not saying that chicken soup will *cure* a cold. There is no real cure for the cold virus. You just have to let it run its course, and the best you can do is treat the symptoms. What we *are* saying is that chicken soup does help with at least one of the annoying symptoms of a cold.

Sipping chicken soup can help relieve clogged nasal passages. Whether it's in the taste or the smell, no one is sure, but taking a cup of hot chicken soup helps loosen the mucus and lets you blow your nose more easily. In fact, researchers at Mount Sinai Medical Center in Miami discovered that chicken soup had ingredients that allowed mucus to flow more freely. (Strangely enough, the researchers couldn't say exactly what it was.) A running nose may make you sneeze more or blow your nose more often, and these are two ways to help relieve the symptoms of a cold.

In a small way, soup also helps by adding more fluids into your system. Drinking water and other clear liquids is a way to avoid dehydration, which is a result of having a fever.

So your mother was right after all. You got a cold? Have some chicken soup. It'll help.

It couldn't hurt.

WATER BOILS FASTER WHEN YOU ADD SALT

....

"We boil at different degrees."
RALPH WALDO EMERSON, *SOCIETY AND SOLITUDE*, "ELOQUENCE"

There we were fixing up a big pot of pasta, waiting for the water to boil, when a familiar voice was heard. Yep, it was the old wives with some more wisdom. They said that it's ridiculous to wait so long for water to boil. All we needed to do was add some salt and pretty soon there would be bubbles aplenty. After all, anyone who knows anything about cooking pasta puts salt in the water first.

We decided to check first with some of these pasta experts. And it's true that they all add salt to water before it boils. However, none of them really knew why they did this. Most assumed it had something to do with taste, but others agreed with the old wives and said, yes, it did make the water boil more quickly.

Ignoring our hunger, we decided to get a scientific explanation once and for all. We consulted Laura Bosworth Bucher, a metallurgical engineer. She said that no, water does not boil faster when you add salt. She explained that when you add salt to water it becomes a solution, and in this particular case, water by itself has a lower boiling point than the solution. So if you had two pots the same size with the same amount of water and added salt to one and put them both over the exact same heat, the pure water would reach its boiling point more quickly.

Ms. Bucher went on to say, though, that there *is* a practical reason to add salt to the water when cooking pasta. Because the water takes longer to boil, more heat is needed to bring the water to a boil. This, in turn, means that salted water boils at a higher temperature than plain water. Therefore, pasta cooks more quickly in salted water because the water is hotter. So adding the salt might save you time after all, but not in the way you thought.

She also discussed the fact that some people also add olive oil to the water. This has no effect on the boiling point, Ms. Bucher said, because oil and water do not mix. The oil stays on top and the two do not become chemically bonded.

There may also be what you could call psychological reasons why people think salt makes water boil faster. When you add the salt, it falls through the water and dissolves. This looks very similar to the small bubbles that signal the onset of boiling. So people may think that the water is boiling while actually it's just becoming salty.

So while this tale is not true, it's still a good idea to add salt to the water if you're making pasta. Of course, if your blood pressure is high, you might want to hold the salt and wait a few more minutes for dinner to be ready.

SHOCK CAN TURN YOUR HAIR WHITE
OVERNIGHT

··

"Then a spirit passed before my face; the hair of my flesh stood up."
JOB 4:15

This is one of those stories that everyone's heard. A friend swears that a friend of a friend had a horrible incident—they either saw the ghost of their long-dead grandmother, came face-to-face with a grizzly, or barely survived a plane crash. The next day the friend of a friend's hair had turned white. They had been so frightened that the color was scared right out of their hair.

As if scientists don't have enough to do, there have been no studies that show that this has ever happened or that it is even possible. There are diseases that can speed up the graying process or make one's hair lose color at an early age. There are also people whose hair, for genetic reasons, turns gray relatively early in life. Since this is not "normal" we tend to feel the need to attach a more logical reason to its occurrence. How the shock-white hair connection started isn't clear, but it works for some.

The image we have of someone's being *really* scared is of a terrified face beneath a head of hair standing straight up. This actually has roots in reality. You've heard of people being so frightened that the hair on the back of their neck stands straight up. Well, when we get cold or really scared, we get goose bumps. In medical terms, goose bumps are the result of the contraction of the erector pili muscles. Some animals are able to make their hair stand up straight as a defense mechanism—it makes them look bigger. Humans have the same reaction, although it only shows as bumps on our skin.

So, in a way, our hair does stand up when we're frightened.

Hair color, though, is caused by the pigment called melanin, which is produced in the cortex of the hair follicle. The shaft of each hair contains this pigment. When hair "turns gray," it's really just that the pigment is no longer being produced, making it appear gray.

So the next time you're face-to-face with a wild animal or see the ghost of the local axe murderer, be scared. Be very scared. But don't worry about the color of your hair.

MICROWAVE OVENS CAN MAKE MEN STERILE

"If you can't stand the heat, get out of the kitchen."
HARRY S. TRUMAN

Since they were first introduced, microwave ovens have been accused of causing cancer and a wide range of other physical ailments including sterility. Here was a new invention that seemed as though it literally cooked by magic. It didn't get hot, there was no need for those big oven mitts, and food could be cooked in a fraction of the usual time. Anything that magical had to have a strange effect on humans, right?

So the fear of microwave ovens is really quite understandable. You put a glass of water into a box, push a button, and with no external source of heat, the water boils. The area around whatever you're heating doesn't even get hot, unlike regular ovens. Using an external source of heat cooks food from the outside in; microwaves cook food from the inside out by exciting water molecules with an electrical field. It's when these molecules become excited and agitated that their friction causes heat, thus cooking food from within. The containers used in microwave cooking don't heat up because they don't absorb microwaves like water molecules do. It's only the heat from the food itself that makes plates and glass cookware warm.

It is true that microwave energy can be dangerous. This is why the U.S. Bureau of Radiological Health has determined strict standards for leakage that all manufacturers of microwave ovens must meet. All doors and locks have one or two attachments that act as backups to ensure that no microwaves escape. Still, *Consumer Reports* suggests standing several feet away from the oven while it's on just to be safe.

It's thought by some that microwaves and their way of cooking can "cook" a man to sterility. It is true that one cause of a lower sperm count is an elevated temperature, which is why testicles are located outside of a man's body and why they have a half degree lower temperature. So, the reasoning goes that microwave ovens can raise the temperature enough to make a man sterile.

This may just be an excuse for a guy to get out of making dinner. It's a creative excuse, but not legitimate. If your oven meets all the requirements set forth for manufacturers, no leakage should occur. Plus, once the oven door is opened, there are no "leftover" waves that can shoot out. Once the oven's off, it's off. Also, there are no microwaves in the food itself or in the container in which it was cooked. To put it simply, the food has not become "radioactive."

Microwave ovens today are built to rigorous standards and are checked carefully for leakage. If you have an older oven, then obviously the technology and safety features will not be as up-to-date. But the chances of microwave leakage from even those older ovens is minimal. Still, it's a good idea to stand back from a microwave oven whenever it's in use no matter how old it is. But will microwave ovens make men sterile? That's just something the old wives cooked up.

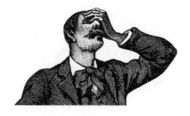

A "HAIR OF THE DOG" WILL HELP A HANGOVER

*"You take one down, pass it around,
ninety-nine bottles of beer on the wall."*
TRADITIONAL SONG

What a night. You really outdid yourself this time. You're not sure where you were, you're not sure how you got home, and you certainly don't remember how the name "Ginger" got tattooed on your arm. (You don't even know a Ginger.) All you know is that you're barely alive. Your head hurts, your stomach aches, even your name feels lousy. What can you possibly take to feel better? A friend quietly suggests a hair of the dog.

For those unfamiliar with this saying, no, it doesn't mean swallowing that which Rover has shed. The complete saying is "a hair of the dog that bit you," meaning that the best way to get over the effects of a night of drinking a particular alcoholic beverage (the dog) is to have another drink of the same (the hair) the next morning.

This tale has its roots in the Middle Ages. In those days, one common way to treat a dog bite was to take a few hairs from the offending pooch and put them on the wound. Years later, those curative hairs have become a metaphor for how to treat overindulging. And we do refer to a strong drink as having a good "bite" to it.

But will a little "hair of the dog" help your hangover? Yes and no, mostly no. A drink may make you feel better temporarily because alcohol does have a sedative effect on the jittery nerves that accompany a hangover, but then you're just continuing the same vicious cycle that led to the hangover in the first place.

When you drink alcohol you lose salt, water, potassium, and other elements. Replacing these elements may help treat the effects of overindulging, such as headaches, nausea, etc. Since alcohol is a diuretic, drinking a lot of fluids will help remedy the dehydration caused by the alcohol. Eating (if you can stand to) will also help because it will raise your metabolic rate. Soup and coffee can also do you some good.

But the only real cure for a hangover is time. Your body needs time to recover from the effects of alcohol. While fluids and food might help some of the effects, it's much easier to prevent hangovers than treat them. Eating before you drink can slow the effects of alcohol, and the more slowly you drink, the less drastic the effects. But moderation is the key. Of course, not drinking at all is the best way to avoid a hangover altogether.

If you've ever awakened the morning after with a hangover, another drink is probably the last thing you wanted. In those first few moments, it might even seem more appealing to literally *put* a few of Rover's clippings in your mouth.

DON'T SWALLOW CHEWING GUM BECAUSE IT'LL NEVER DIGEST

"Give me a good digestion, Lord
And also something to digest."
Anonymous, "A Pilgrim's Grace"

This warning makes the rounds on the playground of nearly every elementary school. It's been said by boys playing catch on the ball field and by girls running together on their way home from school. It's probably been around since, well, since the ancient Greeks began chewing gum made from the resin of spruce trees. (It also belongs to the wives' tales category that includes the undeniable fact that if you swallow a watermelon seed a watermelon will grow in your stomach.)

The "logic" behind not swallowing gum is based on a couple of observations made by nearly every boy and girl.

If you've ever blown a bubble that popped and stuck to every inch of your face, you already know the first one. Gum is sticky and therefore might get caught somewhere in your digestive system and never come out, perhaps causing irreparable damage. What some people (old wives included) fail to realize is that the inside of our bodies is not like the outside (be grateful). Once in the mouth, gum is surrounded by saliva; gum never sticks to your tongue, right? And if swallowed there is no chance that it will stick inside your stomach or intestines because of the acids and the lining.

The second observation is that chewing gum doesn't dissolve in your mouth. Actually, it is true that gum cannot be digested. Until the 1940s, gum was made from the sap of the sapodilla tree, called chicle (hence the name Chicklets), but it's now manufactured using chemicals and, believe it or not, petroleum by-products. So, if you swallow that stick of gum, it won't break down in your stomach. Neither will it stay there forever. It may take a few days, but it will eventually pass naturally.

So don't worry about a piece of gum sitting in your stomach for the rest of your life. This is not, of course, an invitation to swallow gum. But if you do, it will not get caught on the watermelon patch that's probably growing inside of you.

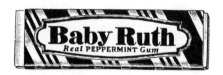

TILT YOUR HEAD BACK TO STOP A NOSEBLEED

Whether or not it's due to our brother's hitting us in the face with a football, we've all experienced nosebleeds. And when this happens, there's always one person in the crowd who tells you to tilt your head back to stop the bleeding. Usually this is the person who passes out at the sight of blood.

And this would seem to make sense because tilting back your head won't stop the bleeding but it will stop the blood from coming out of your nose. The question is, if the blood doesn't come out of your nose, where does it go? In this case it might go down your throat, causing you to choke and have a bigger problem than just a bloody nose.

Whatever the cause, nosebleeds are the result of blood vessels breaking in the nose. According to Dr. Henry Harris at the Albert Einstein School of Medicine, quoted in *Ladies' Home Journal,* most nosebleeds happen in the front part of the wall between our nostrils called the septum. Some people think that the blood in a nosebleed actually comes from somewhere else and just uses the nose as a convenient exit. Most nosebleeds, however, are caused by a blow to the nose or by blowing your nose too much because of a cold or allergies. Also, nosebleeds happen more frequently in winter when the nasal tissues are drier and we tend to blow our noses more often.

Because the bleeding actually comes from the nose, the best way to stop a nosebleed is to apply pressure. In fact, it's better to lean *forward,* not back, to be sure not to swallow any blood. Then pinch your nostrils together to help the blood to clot more quickly and to stop the blood from running all over your shirt. (Boxers, you'll notice, shove cotton swabs up their noses to stop bleeding during a fight. This is a little less attractive, but when you're trying to bloody someone else's nose, looks aren't the first thing on your mind.)

Some people also believe that applying pressure to the lip beneath the nose helps stop a nosebleed because you cut off the blood supply. Actually, that does cut down on it, but direct pressure is the only real way to stop bleeding.

OATMEAL BATHS ARE BEST FOR POISON IVY

"Try these delicious serving ideas . . ." QUAKER OATS

"Dear Mom and Dad,

Camp is great. So far I've made twelve lanyards in crafts and I've almost learned to paddle a canoe. The other day we went on a hike in the woods. It was fun, but when I got back to the cabin I had this itch . . ."

We all know what comes next. Little Johnny starts scratching his arm and pretty soon that rash spreads to his side and his back and his legs, and eventually he's one large blister. Now *there's* something to write home about.

Once exposed to urushiol, the chemical in poison ivy (and poison oak) that produces the allergic reaction, it usually takes twenty-four to forty-eight hours for the exposed area to begin to blister. Over 100 million people in the United States are allergic to it. That's a lot of kids in a lot of camps.

There are also a number of cures that have been recommended down through the years, some chemical, some herbal, and some, disgusting. Some of the more unusual treatments include meat tenderizer, ammonia, paint thinner, and horse urine. Yes, horse urine.

In case you don't live near a stable, one of the more common suggestions is to take an oatmeal bath. Technically speaking, this is an old wives' tale that is completely true. But it may not be what you think.

When most people hear about taking an oatmeal bath they think they can fill up their bathtub and pour in a few of those round boxes of oatmeal with the quaker on the label, plus whatever's left over from breakfast. Oatmeal baths *are* sometimes recommended, but it is colloidal oatmeal that is used, not the everyday-heat-and-serve-makes-you-feel-good-inside-add-a-little-cinnamon oatmeal. This particular type of oatmeal is found at the pharmacy, not in the cereal aisle at the grocery store. What colloidal oatmeal does is dry up the blisters once they start oozing so the healing process can begin. Be sure to rinse it all off, though. Dried oatmeal will only make your skin itch more!

While you can take an oatmeal bath, some people simply apply the mixture with a washcloth to whatever part of the body happens to be infected. This is sometimes the preferred method since, as you might imagine, an oatmeal bath leaves more than a ring around the tub.

The best way to deal with poison ivy is to avoid it altogether. Learn what it looks like and just stay away. The old adage, "Leaves of three, let them be" may be another old wives' tale, but it is also sound medical advice. However, if Johnny comes back from camp with a familiar red glow, an oatmeal bath might be just the thing.

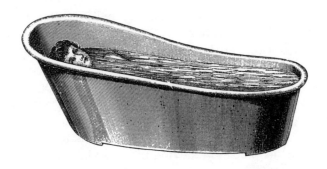

WEARING COPPER JEWELRY IS GOOD FOR ARTHRITIS

"Gold is for the mistress—silver for the maid—
Copper for craftsman cunning at his trade."
RUDYARD KIPLING, "COLD IRON"

Almost 50 million people in the United States alone suffer from arthritis. And it's not just older folks who have it. Children, professional athletes, and young adults alike complain about that pain and stiffness in their hands and joints. Even dogs can have arthritis.

Most arthritis sufferers take aspirin or other painkillers to help alleviate their pain. Some, though, swear by the healing powers of copper. In whatever form—copper rings, copper bracelets—copper is said to provide real relief for arthritis sufferers.

There actually is a more scientific reason for wearing copper. Copper is one of the elements our body needs. Studies show, however, that people who have trouble absorbing copper suffer more frequently from arthritis pain. This means that neither eating foods containing copper nor taking copper supplements can provide the arthritis sufferer with increased levels of copper in their system.

Hence the rings and bracelets. It's believed that wearing copper jewelry is another way to get the copper you need. Dr. Helmar Dollwet, in his book *The Copper Bracelet and Arthritis,* says, "The dissolved copper from a bracelet bypasses the oral route by entering the body through the skin." He goes on to say that studies have proven that the body uses copper to deal with pain.

Most doctors are suspicious, though. While they agree that copper has its place in relieving pain and inflammation on a metabolic level, how it's introduced into the body is another question. Many think that changing the diet is the best way to get more copper. Others, though, don't completely dismiss wearing copper bracelets and rings. If they make a patient feel better, there's no reason for them to stop wearing them, one physician said.

In a way, then, the old wives' tale was right about this one. So the next time Rover complains about his achin' back in the morning, you might want to try a nice copper dog collar or paw bracelet. Keeping it on him is another thing.

USING ANTIPERSPIRANT CAN LEAD TO ALZHEIMER'S DISEASE

"Old age should burn and rave at close of day;
Rage, rage against the dying of the light."
DYLAN THOMAS, "DO NOT GO GENTLE INTO THAT GOOD NIGHT"

Researchers are still debating the cause of this terrible disease, both in terms of how one is afflicted and how the disease works on the genetic level.

Alzheimer's disease was only recently discovered. It's now believed that many recorded cases of senility or dementia throughout history may in fact have been Alzheimer's disease. The causes of the disease have been thought to be everything from tea kettles to boxing. It's only with recent developments in genetic research that a true understanding has begun.

The link between deodorants and Alzheimer's disease is a key ingredient in most antiperspirants: aluminum. It has been commonly thought that there is a definite relationship between aluminum and Alzheimer's disease. Many believe that foods cooked in aluminum pots might cause Alzheimer's disease, and one recent study suggested that even drinking water treated with aluminum sulfate (used at many municipal water treatment plants) could be a contributing factor.

But even experts in medical research aren't sure about the connection between aluminum and Alzheimer's disease. A 1993 study at the University of California at Berkeley found that a link between aluminum and Alzheimer's disease was inconclusive. In fact, Alzheimer's may be a genetic disease. Researchers at Duke University Medical Center found that four-fifths of Alzheimer's cases studied were due to a defect in the code of a single gene. In other words, the development of the disease may be hereditary and may not have viral or environmental origins.

So whether your roll-on might contribute to the chances of your developing Alzheimer's disease, no one really knows for sure. If you want to play it safe, look for those deodorants that do not contain aluminum. (It was also found that cooking foods in aluminum pots versus iron or steel pots does increase the amount of aluminum in the food by over five hundred times, but, again, there is still no proven link between more aluminum in the diet and getting Alzheimer's disease.)

As medical research progresses, we learn more and more about Alzheimer's disease, but we still don't know what causes it. Antiperspirants and aluminum may have no connection to the disease at all. It is thought, though, that a breakthrough in determining what causes Alzheimer's disease is not too far in the future.

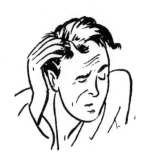

RUB A POTATO ON YOUR FACE AND HANDS TO SOFTEN THE SKIN

....

"You like PO-TA-TO and I like PO-TAH-TO . . ."
GEORGE AND IRA GERSHWIN, "LET'S CALL THE WHOLE THING OFF"

Okay, now close your eyes and try to picture Cindy Crawford and her fellow supermodels with a spud in their hands, rubbing their million-dollar cheeks for that softer-than-soft feeling. Does this make sense to you?

There's a reason why you won't find potatoes in the cosmetics section. It's the same reason you won't find chewing gum in the hardware section. Occasionally, everyone uses gum to make something stick right? Well, while you might use gum to temporarily fasten two things together, that only works until the gum dries out. The key word here is "temporarily." A nail or tape is what you need to do the job right.

It's the same with potatoes. When you rub a potato on your hands they feel softer. What you're feeling isn't softer skin, really, but starch. A thin layer comes off the potato when you rub it on your face, on your legs, or on the kitchen counter.

Does this make your skin softer? It makes your skin feel softer to the touch, yes, but it's not the skin you're feeling. It's the starch. However, the thin, smooth film of starch dries out relatively quickly and, left to harden, makes your skin even itchier. It certainly doesn't last like the high-priced skin softeners back in the cosmetics section. So, if you do see Cindy Crawford holding a potato, you can bet she's getting paid a lot of money by Ore-Ida.

Spuds are great for dinner, though. Just keep those french fries off your face.

VITAMIN C PREVENTS COLDS

"A day without orange juice is like a day without sunshine."
ANITA BRYANT

Everyone has an opinion about vitamins. Some are true believers, some gave up taking vitamins when they ate their last fruit-flavored chewable as a child. And vitamin C is one about which opinions are divided not only among the general public, but among those in the medical profession as well.

Try telling anyone who regularly takes vitamin C that it doesn't make a difference. Those who swear by it insist that they get fewer colds than most people and that a few thousand milligrams perks them up whenever they feel a cold coming on. They say that taking vitamin C pills (ascorbic acid) does far more for them than simply drinking orange juice could ever do.

This much is true. But how much vitamin C does the body need?

The Recommended Dietary Allowance (U.S. RDA) of vitamin C is 60 milligrams. (The RDA of any vitamin is based on how much of a particular nutrient is needed to maintain good health in the average healthy person.) The average American diet contains about 72 milligrams of vitamin C, but you can also reach the RDA by drinking half a glass of orange juice. We actually only use 10 milligrams of the recommended 60 milligrams of vitamin C per day; our body stores the other 50 milligrams just in case we miss a day or two.

So how much vitamin C is too much? This is where even the doctors differ. Some feel that the hype over vitamin C's powers of prevention is just that—hype. They point out that if you have extremely high cholesterol, too much vitamin C can increase your risk of heart attack. They also argue that too much of one vitamin can disrupt the balance in your body's complicated chemical makeup. They also point out that the body can only absorb so much C, and that most of it passes through the body anyway.

Advocates of vitamin C point out that the vitamin's benefits can be traced back to the 1500s, when seafaring explorers were discovering the New World . . . and scurvy. British sailors a few centuries later found that the best remedy for scurvy was oranges, lemons, and limes. Hence, the start of the vitamin C craze.

The best known advocate of Vitamin C is Dr. Linus Pauling, whose book *Vitamin C and the Common Cold* set off a run on vitamin stores. In the book, Dr. Pauling suggested that massive doses of ascorbic acid could prevent colds. He said that while individual needs vary, people should take one to three *grams* every day (again, the daily minimum requirement is 60 *milli*grams.) Some researchers said that while vitamin C might not prevent a cold, it can certainly hasten its departure.

Whether it's scurvy or the common cold, the bottom line is that doctors are not in agreement about the benefits of mega-doses of vitamin C. Some say that a normal diet should suffice. Others counter that no diet is always normal (or normally prepared) and that supplements could help.

So we defer to an old wife's advice: Check with your doctor before taking any supplement. And drink your orange juice.

A BABY BORN WITH A CAUL OVER ITS FACE HAS SPECIAL POWERS

....

"That's it, baby. When you got it, flaunt it"
MEL BROOKS IN *THE PRODUCERS*

While in the womb of its mother, a baby is surrounded by a thin membrane filled with amniotic fluid sometimes referred to as a caul. In the vast majority of births, the membrane ruptures and the mother's "water breaks."

21

Sometimes, though, the caul remains intact over the baby's head. When this happens it's often said that the baby was born with a mask. In the days of spells and charms, an event like this took on special importance.

There are many ancient superstitions about being born with a caul, nearly all positive. The most common is that the baby would have good luck, more specifically that he would never die by drowning. (This was undoubtedly related to the protection the caul provided the baby as it floated in the womb, surrounded by amniotic fluid.) In fact, many people would save the caul, and if the baby grew up and traveled by ship, the ship itself would be protected by the power of the caul.

This good luck was ensured provided the caul was saved. If the baby was born with such a mask and it was thrown out, the luck went out with it. The superstition included numerous stories where mothers threw away the cauls after their child reached a certain age, only to have the child drown shortly after. It was also believed that bad luck or a short life was ensured for the baby if the caul were black.

In fact, so strong was the belief in the positive powers of cauls that people would buy and sell them. Sailors especially would seek out midwives from whom they could buy cauls to accompany them on their voyage. Protection from drowning wasn't the only advantage provided by the caul. Other good qualities that resulted from being born with or owning a caul were freedom from curses, eloquence, and general happiness.

In reality, the caul provides protection for the baby before birth. Being born with a caul intact isn't really common, but it's not extraordinary either and it has no effect on the child or the mother. So as far as special powers go, there aren't any here. Something different certainly does happen during the birth, but there's no reason to think that a baby born with a caul would survive the seven seas more easily than one born without.

REDHEADS HAVE TERRIBLE TEMPERS

....

"It's my rule never to lose me temper till it would be detrimental to keep it."
SEAN O'CASEY, *THE PLOUGH AND THE STARS*

We went to the source for this one. When asked about this adage, a redheaded friend couldn't believe her ears. "It's the 1990s and people still say that? You've got to be kidding!" She then stomped angrily out of the room.

The notion that anyone with the nickname "Red" or "Carrottop" would genetically have a worse temper than most comes from the same source that says that anyone with the nickname "Blondie" has trouble spelling her last name.

There are two aspects of human behavior at work here. First, studies show that hair color is one of the first things we notice about a person—height, weight, and age are the others. After all, when an all-points bulletin is put out on the guy who just robbed the bank, isn't hair color one of the characteristics listed? (Okay, unless he's wearing panty hose over his head.)

Second is the associations we bring to the color of that hair. Red is the color of passion. (Try to find a valentine card that doesn't have red in it.) Flames are red. And what color does a bullfighter wave in front of his foe to incite snorts of anger and stampedes of rage?

When people get angry their faces turn red. This is because when we get excited, more blood rushes to the vessels underneath the skin of the face. Since redheads tend to have paler skin, the flushed redness stands out more than with brunettes or blondes. So while everyone turns red when they're angry, it appears that redheads get even more so because their reaction is naturally more noticeable.

Because of their hair color, redheads have faced many misconceptions. It was once believed that doctors could diagnose illnesses solely by the patient's complexion. When people were too red in the face, they were thought to have "ill blood." Therefore, those with red hair must have even more of that bad blood in them. There is another theory (agreed to by many redheads) that people were suspicious of those with red hair purely out of jealousy.

Redheads have been the focus of attention throughout history. Egyptians sometimes ceremonially burned maidens with red hair to rid their country of bad luck. In the Middle Ages, having red hair was a sure sign of witchery. Here, too, the unlucky redhead was burned at the stake. In certain cultures it's believed that having red hair makes you a good conversationalist.

Red hair is acquired genetically. It's caused by pigmentation in the hair (or, sometimes, a quick dye job), not by any type of blood or evil spirits. And pigments are not the cause of bad tempers. What makes for a short fuse? Upbringing and environment, mostly, neither of which have much to do with one's natural hair color.

Now don't get us wrong. Some redheads *do* have bad tempers. And some blondes *do* have trouble spelling their last names. Of course, there are also Benedictine monks who have red hair. The fact is, there aren't any real constant characteristics that go along with hair color. (Sorry, guys, baldness won't make you smarter.)

Hopefully, this will serve as an apology to the above-mentioned redheaded friend, and, if she ever cools down enough to read this, maybe she'll forgive us.

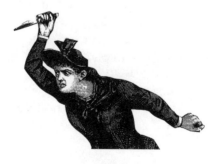

BREAKING A MIRROR MEANS SEVEN YEARS OF BAD LUCK

*"The mirror crack'd from side to side:
'The curse is come upon me,' cried the Lady of Shalott."*
ALFRED, LORD TENNYSON, "THE LADY OF SHALOTT"

What's the worst time of the day? For many it's when you stagger out of bed, struggle to open your eyes, shield them against the sudden light in the bathroom, and take that first look in the mirror. At that moment, the mirror is our worst enemy.

For some, the mirror can be a source of great pleasure; for others, great disappointment. Some say that this is because it makes us confront ourselves. Others who are less philosophical and more narcissistic say the mirror is their best friend. If there is one thing we all know about a mirror, though, it's that a mirror can provide us with one of the easiest ways to turn our luck bad for seven years, no matter what you look like.

Why is this so? When man first stood erect and saw his reflection in a pool of water, he thought, "Surely that can't be me." But then as he moved, he saw his reflection move also. Hmm. He then reasoned that since it wasn't his body, it must be a reflection of his soul. (This is also true of a person's shadow, the source of other old wives' tales.) Since his soul was there in the water, primitive man thought, then as long as the reflection was unharmed, his soul would be fine.

Societies from then on gave special meaning to a person's reflection, and this is where many of the superstitions dealing with mirrors began. Some believe that if you look in a mirror and don't see your reflection, you are dead. Some mothers won't let their babies look in a mirror until a certain age to ensure normal growth. An African tribe believed that if you look into a muddy pool of water, the darkness might steal your reflected soul.

The root of all these beliefs is that a mirror that holds our reflection holds a part of us. So, if that mirror is broken, then part of us will be harmed as well. Make sense? But why seven years? The seven years is based on the fear of that number. Seven is either a very lucky number for some or a very bad number. (See "The Human Body Renews Itself Every Seven Years" for a more detailed discussion about the number seven.)

What the old wives didn't mention, though, was that the only meaning to be attached to breaking a mirror is, perhaps, clumsiness. The biggest danger might just be the broken pieces of glass you forget to pick up. Of course, if you looked like some of those old wives, you might think it bad luck to look in a mirror whether it breaks or not.

NEVER LIGHT THREE ON A SINGLE MATCH

"Come on, baby, light my fire."
JIM MORRISON, "LIGHT MY FIRE"

Here's the way this one works. Let's say you're at a party and you step out for a cigarette with two friends. One of you strikes a match and lights your smoke. You then politely offer the flame to the next person. You then hold the match out for the third person, who quickly blows it out. Why?

Legend has it that the third person to use a match will be saddled with bad luck or even killed soon (which, come to think of it, is pretty bad luck). There are even some who say that all three people sharing the match will meet a terrible fate. As if smoking weren't bad enough.

It's believed by some that this tale started in the Boer War. When soldiers in the trenches would smoke at night, it was a common warning that if you were to keep a match lit long enough to light three cigarettes, the enemy sharpshooters would have enough time to focus their aim and shoot, more than likely at the third person because he'd be the one who held the match last. Bad luck indeed. This story was repeated to us in a slightly different version by an Italian friend, who said the warning about keeping a match lit in wartime started in Italy in World War I as a safeguard against snipers and mortar shells.

However, the true root of this saying has as much to do with the number three as it does with the light from the match. The number three is associated with the Holy Trinity and has a special significance with religious faith and ceremonies. This religious connection is further supported by some who feel the saying began during the Crimean War. Russian soldiers were being held in British POW camps and the British noticed that, during the Russian funeral services, only an ordained clergyman was allowed to light the three candles on the altar. The British adopted this custom and the belief that it was unholy for a nonclergyman to light three candles with one match.

So while this old wives' tale doesn't ring true all the time, with the number of smokers in the modern world, it might serve us well to remember that even one on a match may be too many when it comes to smoking and your health.

PLANTS IN THE HOUSE MEAN MORE OXYGEN

"Get your room full of good air,
then shut the windows and keep it."
STEPHEN LEACOCK, *LITERARY LAPSES*, "HOW TO LIVE TO BE 200"

Let's go back to fifth-grade science class on this one. We all learned that when humans or any other animals breathe, oxygen goes in. When we exhale, carbon dioxide comes out. In with the good, out with the bad.

We also learned that plants do the opposite. When they

"breathe," carbon dioxide goes in and oxygen goes out. This is why they say it's healthy for plants if you talk to them. This way they get their carbon dioxide straight from you and you get oxygen right back from them. Sounds like a pretty convenient relationship, yes?

It actually gets a little more complicated than this, but, yes, having plants in the house does mean more oxygen. This comes as good news to those who know that extra oxygen often means more energy. But, like everything else in life, that's not the whole story.

To say that plants give off oxygen implies that there's going to be a noticeable difference, as though having ferns and violets spread around the room would be similar to being inside an oxygen tent. However, the amount of oxygen released by plants is so minimal that you'd need to turn your living room into a greenhouse to notice any difference.

There is another old wives' tale that goes along with plants and oxygen. It is thought by some that the plants should be removed at night from the room of a bedridden person. This is based on a scientific discovery that reported that plants reverse their "breathing" in the dark, that they take in oxygen and release carbon dioxide. This means that at night they would deprive the patient of needed, healthy air.

A researcher in England in the 1770s was the first to find out that plants release oxygen. A Dutch scientist later found that this was the result of how plants process and save sugar. During the day, plants store sugar, then at night, when they need energy that they can't get from the sun, they use the stored sugar. And they use oxygen to burn the sugar. Therefore, at night they "breathe" oxygen. But, again, the amount of oxygen used at night by a few plants makes no difference to a human.

So while moving your plants from one room to another throughout the day and night certainly has a clear scientific basis, the results aren't anything you'll notice. But at least you can take pride in still being able to remember what you learned in fifth grade.

IF YOU LOSE TEN POUNDS YOU'LL GAIN IT BACK

···

"Outside every fat man there was an even fatter man trying to close in."
KINGSLEY AMIS, *ONE FAT ENGLISHMAN*

If you've ever tried to lose a few pounds, the experience is very familiar. You diet. No more chocolate mousse desserts or extra large buttered popcorns or cookies-and-cream breakfasts. You exercise. You actually walk up two flights of steps instead of using the elevator. The clothes aren't hung on the stationary bike anymore. And after what seems to be an eternity of austerity you reach your goal: Ten pounds are gone and you look and feel great.

And before you know it . . . it's baaaack! No matter how much you tried, no matter how much you kept to your original diet, you always seemed to gain back the weight you lost.

The explanation used to be simple. "You gained back the ten pounds? Oh, that's just an old wives' tale," the critics would say. "You just got lazy or hungry and went back to your old ways and *that's* why you gained back the weight. Now quit complaining."

Well, believe it or not, medical science has come to the rescue of the old wives on this one.

In a recent discovery at the New York Obesity Research Center at Rockefeller University, scientists found that the human body tries to keep itself at its original, pre-diet weight. Once the body senses that you've lost weight, it slows down your metabolism, which is the amount of energy you need to breathe, burn calories, digest food, keep your heart beating, etc. The body also makes your muscles work more efficiently. This means that you'll burn fewer calories doing work or exercising at the new, lower weight than you did at your original weight. Depressing as it sounds, what this means is that once you've lost that first ten pounds, you'll have to work harder and eat even less to maintain the weight loss, otherwise you'll slowly return to where you were before.

A study published in the *New England Journal of Medicine* says that if you don't exercise once you've lost weight, you have to cut down on your calories 15 percent more than doctors previously thought. For example, a man who always weighed 165 and lost 10 pounds to weigh 155 would have to eat 15 percent fewer calories to maintain that weight than a man who always weighed 155.

This means that once you drop a few pounds you'll still have to drink even fewer milkshakes and climb even more stairs to maintain your weight loss. Just when you were feeling proud of yourself, your body tries to gain weight back for you.

It's not fair. It really isn't.

OPENING AN UMBRELLA INDOORS WILL BRING BAD LUCK

....

"All men are equal—all men, that is to say, who possess umbrellas."
E. M. FORSTER, *HOWARD'S END*

Everyone's heard this one, so it must be true, right?
Wrong.
Now don't get us wrong. Opening an umbrella indoors very well could bring you bad luck if you're not careful. In fact, this superstition began in the first place because of how umbrellas were originally built. They operated pretty much the same way as they do today, but umbrellas were once made with springs that were rather primitive. Because they were so stiff, the springs would open the umbrellas quite suddenly and uncontrollably. And if you were indoors, the chances of acci-

dentally knocking over the nearest breakable were quite good.

But, of course, common sense can't be the only reason not to open an umbrella indoors. So, people started assigning other, more mystical dangers to this act. Some believe that an umbrella opened indoors is an invitation for rain. Others think that if you open your umbrella in a friend's house, you're showing disrespect for the worthiness of that person's roof.

Umbrella superstitions also came from China and Africa, where parasols were used to shade people from the sun, which umbrellas eventually came to symbolize. The sun represented a higher power in those countries, so it was sacrilegious to use umbrellas in an inappropriate way, which would mean opening one inside a house. Also, clergymen were among the first to use umbrellas, so that was another religious element attached to them.

Today, however, the umbrella is used mainly for protection from rain. The religious symbolism isn't commonly known. The fact is, not a lot of people know why it's supposed to be bad luck to open an umbrella indoors. It just is.

However, if it makes you feel any better, there is really no reason to open an umbrella indoors anyway. Unless, of course, your roof is leaking. In that case, your luck was bad before you opened the umbrella.

BALDNESS IS HEREDITARY

"Who loves you, baby?"
TELLY SAVALAS (AS LIEUTENANT THEO KOJAK) *KOJAK*

Grass doesn't grow on a busy street. Baldness is a sign of virility. Patrick Stewart is cool.

Despite all these proclamations, losing one's hair is the biggest fear of many men. Samson losing his locks set a precedent that has yet to be overcome. From the wig-wearing fops of the Restoration to present-day hair weave studs, men have always equated personal worth with how much or how little hair they have.

Doctors are a little more realistic. "Having hair isn't necessarily an issue of vanity; it's an issue of being comfortable in society," said Dr. Dowling Stough, a clinical assistant professor of dermatology at the University of Arkansas, in *Better Homes and Gardens*. It's only natural to want to keep what we've got.

Losing one's hair isn't the greatest experience for men (or women, for that matter). Over the years people have theorized that everything from worrying too much to wearing hats can cause you to lose your hair. The speculation has gone from the ridiculous to the, well, more ridiculous. And it's odd that the old wives would chime in with a relatively scientific theory: genetics.

And they're right. It's true. Heredity is the cause of male pattern baldness, the most common type of balding. It can be inherited from either your father's or mother's side. It can also affect women, usually causing thin hair. (True baldness doesn't happen too often to women, but it's not impossible.)

"Bunk," you say. Your sister was pregnant last year and lost some hair, and just recently your cousin had major surgery and came out with less hair than he went in with.

True, there are other causes of hair loss. According to the American Academy of Dermatology, almost two-thirds of all men and women deal with some form of hair loss or thinning. There are many causes: not getting enough protein in the diet, certain medications, childbirth, birth control pills, chemotherapy. The hair loss is sometimes temporary, sometimes not. There is also a disease called alopecia areata that causes sudden, permanent hair loss, which currently affects about 2.5 million Americans.

So, while there are other causes for losing one's hair, the most common, male pattern balding, is genetic. But don't panic if you notice a few hairs in your comb in the morning. Hair loss is really quite normal. As teenagers, we have about 100,000 hairs on our heads and we shed about 50 to 100 per day. Usually new hair grows in its place, however your head can only have so many hairs on it. Hair grows out of follicles, and the number of follicles on your head never increases. So if you had thin hair when you were young, you'll always have thin hair.

There are new medicines being developed to stimulate hair growth, Minoxidil being the most popular. But these drugs help with thinning hair only. There is no real cure for baldness yet. Some doctors are hopeful, but they add not to be fooled by ads for "miracle hair-growth drugs" because such drugs simply don't exist.

So until a hair pill is developed, you'll just have to live with the pattern of hair growth and loss you inherited. Baldness may be inevitable for some, but, come on, it's nothing to lose your hair over.

THE HUMAN BODY RENEWS ITSELF EVERY SEVEN YEARS

"All the world's a stage,
And all the men and women merely players;
They have their exits and their entrances;
And one man in his time plays many parts,
His acts being seven ages."
WILLIAM SHAKESPEARE, AS YOU LIKE IT

When their kids were young and misbehaving, the old wives never feared because they knew that once a kid reached the age of seven (if they didn't kill him first) he would change for the better. It's been long believed that kids stop being brats as soon as they reach seven. They become new people. Their bodies and their minds go through noticeable changes.

It's further believed that the human body continues to change every seven years. We are reborn in body and mind not only at seven, but at fourteen, twenty-one, twenty-eight, thirty-five, forty-two, forty-nine, and so on. In fact, it was widely believed that when someone reaches sixty-three (another multiple of seven), they would live to a very old age.

Now, chances are that if you're a parent you might have noticed a change in your kids around age seven. Chances are, too, that you noticed some pretty big changes at other ages. The reality is that our bodies are constantly changing. They are not renewed in any way every seven years. The old wives had this one all wrong.

Why seven in the first place? For some reason, this is one of those numbers (like three or thirteen) that always has some significance attached to it. The Bible describes the seven days of creation. Early astrologers knew of only seven heavenly bodies: the Sun, the Moon, Mercury, Venus, Mars, Jupiter, and Saturn. To each of these they assigned a god or goddess whose influence ruled our destinies. Under these influences, our lives were also divided into seven ages. Ancient Greek scientists thought that there were seven substances that made up our bodies. There are seven virtues and seven seas. And we all know what happens after seven years of marriage—the seven-year itch, of course.

Rather than waiting seven years for your body to be rejuvenated, you might want to join a local health club now rather than later. And don't expect your little devil to become angelic once he turns seven. He has a lot of mischief to go through yet.

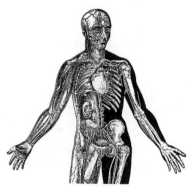

DOGS CAN SENSE FEAR

"Cave canem"
LATIN FOR "BEWARE OF THE DOG"

Every letter carrier's fear is to walk up the path to a house and see Rover with a snarl on his face and hear an attitude in his growl. When we meet a dog in this mood we're told to be perfectly still and not show our fear. They can smell it.

Can they really? Well, maybe. The fact is that animals' senses such as hearing and smell are more finely tuned than our own. They're also capable of sensing chemicals called pheromones. Animals release pheromones to let other animals know that they should stay away or that they're in the mood for love. For animals, pheromones provide a means of communication the same way that verbal language does for humans.

But humans also release physiological signs that they feel a certain way. When we're afraid, we react by sweating. Some people sweat so much that they become drenched, others have only a little perspiration on their upper lip. In either case, our bodies produce chemicals when we're faced with a frightening situation. And dogs are able to perceive these signs with their keener senses.

When we're afraid we also have other reactions, both chemical and physical, some more obvious than others. Our eyes might grow wider, we may shake slightly or utter a brief cry for help. No one really has the ability to mask completely all the reactions we have when we become frightened. So while you try to not let them see you sweat, in reality dogs are perceptive enough to know if we're afraid of them.

For centuries dogs have been thought to have special powers. In some societies, dogs were believed to be able to see ghosts. There are still people today who believe that if you hear a dog howling in the night, it means that someone is dead or is about to die.

This old wives' tale, then, is true. Dogs are able to sense fear because of our physical reactions. If you don't believe us, go by your local post office and ask around.

SPICY FOODS GIVE YOU NIGHTMARES

"In the nightmare of the dark,
all the dogs of Europe bark."
W. H. AUDEN, "IN MEMORY OF W. B. YEATS"

Ever have that craving for a pizza or some of that leftover barbecue during the late show? Ever wake up in the middle of the night and know that you can't get back to sleep unless you raid the refrigerator? Ever dream that you were being chased by a hundred-foot-long reptile breathing fire? Ever swear you'll never eat that stuff before bedtime again?

Don't say you weren't warned. Almost everyone gets a craving for a late-night snack every once in a while, and almost everyone has someone else warning them that eating too late will give them nightmares. Is this true? Are we destined to be chased in our dreams for committing the mere sin of a midnight taco?

Maybe. A few years ago, researchers at St. George's Medical School in London found that what you eat can indeed have an influence on how much you dream. They said that a normal diet will give you a normal night's sleep. And since you dream nearly every night, you'd also have a normal night's worth of dreaming. But your dreams become a lot more active, they found, when you eat a lot of foods that are high in fat or starch. This includes pizza, tacos, and most of those spicy foods you were always warned about.

It was once believed that nightmares were evil spirits trying to crush us while we slept. In fact, that's where the "mare" comes from; the dreams are like a big horse coming to get us. If you've ever tossed all night and awakened in a cold sweat because you dreamed of being chased by hungry dogs in hell, you might feel a little trampled. In reality, though, it probably has more to do with those three chili dogs than any evil spirits. Of course at that point, chili dogs *are* evil.

A WOMAN CAN'T GET PREGNANT WHILE NURSING

"Milk. It does a body good."
ADVERTISING SLOGAN FOR MILK

You and your wife are new parents. You're enjoying the experience so much that you think another baby might be fun, so you bring it up to her. She stares at you, not believing her ears. "Give me a break. I've just given birth and I'm caring for a baby twenty-four hours a day and breast-feeding all hours of the night, and you want to have *another* baby? You've got to be kidding." The subject is closed.

This is probably all the birth control needed in most households with babies. But, exhaustion aside, the question remains: Can you get pregnant while you're nursing? Is breast-feeding an effective method of contraception?

There is actually some truth to this. When women breast-feed they are lactating. Lactation delays a woman's return to ovulation after she's given birth. Breast-feeding cuts down on the hormone needed to keep an egg in the ovaries, thus lowering the chance of getting pregnant. The more a woman breast-feeds her baby (not using other sources of milk) the longer the delay before she starts ovulating again. One report found that if a woman breast-fed her baby and didn't have her period for six months after she gave birth, her chances of conceiving were less than 2 percent.

There are exceptions, of course, so be sure to check with your doctor if you plan to rely on this form of contraception. But, as a rule, this old wives' tale is true. Now as for having another baby while you're still nursing one, you might want to refer to the first *Old Wives' Tales* book and consult the chapter on spinach giving you more strength.

BRUSHING YOUR HAIR AT LEAST ONE HUNDRED STROKES WILL KEEP IT CLEAN

"The Spartans on the sea-wet rock sat down and combed their hair."
A. E. HOUSMAN, "THE ORACLES"

Sure, this is fine for most people, but imagine if Rapunzel had lived by this saying. With hair that long, she'd not only be brushing all day, but by the time she finished her arms would look like Arnold Schwarzeneggar's. We're not sure that prince fellow would have climbed up to see *that*.

Okay, but is this tale true? Well, the old wives weren't all wrong on this one, but then again they weren't all right either.

This practice of brushing your hair one hundred strokes to keep it clean started back in the days when it wasn't convenient or even possible to wash your hair regularly. This was due either to a lack of water or, more likely, to an absence of soap. (In fact, history books don't mention soap until about the first century A.D. The early Greeks and Romans used to bathe in water and scrape their skin with strigils to get clean.)

In reality, the theory was that if you combed your hair enough times, you'd remove any dirt that might be in there. In this regard the saying makes sense. It's just a way of dry-washing your hair.

It can get a bit hairy, though. If you have oily hair, too much brushing takes oil from the scalp to the ends of the hair. Thus, by following the old wives' advice, you'd actually make your hair appear dirtier and less attractive.

However, there was another reason they advised women to brush their hair so many times. In areas where head lice were a problem, one hundred strokes with a comb or brush was the best defense against an all-out infestation. Repeated combing would cut the critters off at the legs and eventually fling them out of a woman's hair.

But why one hundred times? It's a nice, round, large number that would ensure that each of the 150,000 hairs on the average human head would get a workout. It's also a number more magical than, say, eighty-four.

Furthermore, it was believed at one time that brushing the hair one hundred strokes at the end of the day would make it grow longer more quickly. Again, there's a hair of truth here. It's known that massaging the scalp helps to promote hair growth. And unless you're extra careful, chances are that your scalp will make some pretty good contact during one hundred strokes.

Still, the next time you visit your Rapunzel and she looks as though she could beat you at arm wrestling, you might want to suggest a good shampoo and conditioner. Or a trim.

WOMEN ARE MOST INTERESTED IN THE SIZE OF A MAN'S PENIS

"It's not the size of the ship, but the motion of the ocean."
MEN EVERYWHERE

No pun intended, but most men wouldn't touch this old wives' tale with a ten-foot pole. So, we'll have to leave it to women and researchers.

After a random, nonscientific sampling, we found that size is one of the least concerns women have in their sexual partners. Yes, some women think size is important, but it is a myth that a man need have a, well, a ten-foot pole to be an effective lover. Truth be told, in general there is little difference in size, of the penises (when erect) of most men. There are, of course, exceptions. One researcher found that men who are smaller in the unexcited state grow proportionately more than their larger brothers. Therefore, when it matters, differences in size are not that profound.

Still, sex researchers Masters and Johnson found that a woman's vagina adjusts itself during intercourse to the size of the man. This, they say, means that size is not important on either side of the bed. In other words, everything was designed to fit together nicely.

There is no accounting for preference, however. Some women may simply get more pleasure from a man better endowed, just as some men may have a preference in the size of women's attributes. Society does place more emphasis on size, just as it does on slender bodies, perfect skin, and large breasts. Because of this, men are always given solutions to their shortcomings. A random sampling of the *Los Angeles Times* shows several ads for surgical penile enlargement. There are also many home "remedies," which a visit to any high school locker room could provide.

We have no idea how the old husbands of the old wives measured up. Perhaps this tale grew out of the personal preferences of the old wives. Regardless, men throughout the years have felt inadequate and women have been unfairly labeled as being size hungry. But now you know the long and short of it.

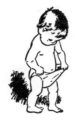

SNEEZING AFTER INTERCOURSE PREVENTS PREGNANCY

··

"Sneeze on a Monday, you sneeze for danger
Sneeze on a Tuesday, you kiss a stranger."
ANONYMOUS FOLKLORE

To the uninformed, this would appear to be nothing more than advice from people who have no idea how the human body works. To the skeptical, this seems to be an irresponsible and baseless lie.

And they would all be right. But let's humor the old wives and see if we can explain how this is supposed to work. Sneezing after sex is believed to jar loose and expel the sperm that the man left behind. Simple.

Believe it or not, some intelligent people used to believe that sneezing prevented pregnancy. In fact, a physician in ancient Greece named Dioscorides thought that since sneezing got rid of the man's sperm, and since pepper could make a woman sneeze, then the best thing to do was to apply the pepper not to the nose but, well, you get the idea. We're not sure that any sneezing was supposed to take place but he believed that pepper had certain healing qualities and would do the trick.

Believe it or not, pepper wasn't the worst thing that was ever prescribed as a contraceptive. Everything from mixtures of parts of the acacia plant and honey to elephant and mouse dung were used. Actually, odd as it may seem, the basic principle was right. All of those concoctions had high levels of lactic acid, which is one of the main ingredients of modern day contraceptive creams.

Unfortunately, preventing pregnancy is not as easy as sneezing. If it were, we suppose saying "Bless you" after a sneeze would take on a whole new meaning. And for those wishful thinkers out there, we hate to disappoint you but this old wives' tale is nowhere near true.

TAKE MILK BATHS FOR GOOD SKIN

"The cow is of the bovine ilk;
one end is moo, the other, milk."
OGDEN NASH, "THE COW"

Cleopatra had it made. Here was a woman who could have any man she wanted and was pampered and had the best beauty treatments available at that time. Picture her there, lying back, eating grapes with a bunch of muscle-heads fanning her. Why? Because she was beautiful enough to start a war over. And what made her so beautiful? What was her secret? We're told that one of her ways of achieving her legendary smooth skin was to take milk baths.

Many people believe that taking a bath in milk does wonders for your skin. It's seen as very exotic and a natural way to make your skin smooth and silky. The old wives believed that milk contained properties that would work miracles on your skin.

So should you tell the milkman to bring an extra twenty gallons next week? A milk bath would probably make you feel good. It looks exotic and the milk will have a cooling, soothing effect on you. But will it do wondrous things for your skin? Most doctors think not.

Doctors, though, don't dispute that milk has some good qualities that can help the skin. Some will advise treating a sunburn with a compress of milk and water. This not only cools the skin, but milk also contains protein that helps restore your skin's normal pH factor. Beauty consultants tell their customers to splash their faces with buttermilk before sleeping to help moisturize their skin.

There's also a history to milk baths. In ancient times it was known (and some still believe today) that the best bath in the world is to immerse yourself in a tub of ass' milk. Yes, ass' milk. As you might suspect, this isn't the most readily available type of milk. A quick survey showed that most 7-Eleven's don't carry a supply of ass' milk.

If you want to take a milk bath, it won't hurt you and may make you feel better. Basically, this is a way to pamper yourself. The cost won't pamper your budget, though, which is why some people resort to milk packs. Then there's the problem of cleaning the tub afterward. Of course, you could always have the bunch of muscle-heads you have fanning you bring along their scrub brushes. Now *that's* living like a queen.

UNDERWATER BIRTH ENSURES BABIES A HAPPY, MORE PEACEFUL LIFE

....

*"There is no cure for birth and death
save to enjoy the interval."*
GEORGE SANTAYANA, *SOLILOQUIES IN ENGLAND AND LATER SOLILOQUIES,*
"WAR SHRINES"

For those of you unfamiliar with the concept, underwater birthing is a form of natural childbirth. When going into labor, the woman steps into a pool or tub of water. In some cases, her family joins her, too. Many women, midwives, doctors, and others will tell you of the many benefits of giving birth underwater. But before we mention them, let's see if this old wives' tale holds any water.

If you read the fine print, it says that being born like this gives the baby a more peaceful *life*. What underwater birthing can do is give the baby and mother a less traumatic *birth*.

Whether the baby goes on to live an equally peaceful life is determined by the child's upbringing, not by the first few seconds after its birth. It's true that trauma at birth can have a lasting effect on the child, but it's also true that some babies born under ideal conditions go on to have less than peaceful lives, and that some babies born the old-fashioned way grow up to have completely peaceful lives. Unfortunately, it takes more than being born in a hot tub to ensure a lifetime of bliss.

And while this type of birth may sound dangerous to some, it's really not. Doctors agree that as long as the baby is brought to the surface of the water in a few seconds, there is little danger of its swallowing water. After all, until the child takes its first breath into its lungs through its mouth, it continues to get oxygen through the umbilical cord, as it has for months within the womb.

People believe the basic benefit of underwater childbirth is that the baby will have a less-rude awakening by being taken from a nice, warm womb into a nice, warm watery environment. It's less traumatic. It's also better for the mother, many doctors say. Women tend to be more relaxed in the early stages of labor when immersed in water. They also report less pain during labor and a quicker, more efficient birth.

So while underwater delivery may ensure a more peaceful birth, the rest of the child's life is up to many other factors. Now, if the kid could spend the rest of his life in a hot tub, then you'd have something.

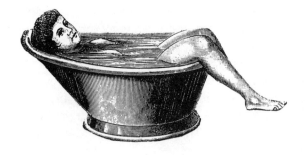

RIDING A HORSE CAN CAUSE A GIRL TO LOSE HER VIRGINITY

···

"Hi-yo Silver, away!"
THE LONE RANGER

There's always been something about a woman's virginity that's held a certain fascination for society. Long ago, it was actually believed that having intercourse with a virgin would cure a man's venereal disease. And we've all heard stories about virgin sacrifices. There were even cultures where, when a man and a woman were married, the king would deflower the girl. It was only after the king was given the gift of the bride that the husband could have his new wife.

A virgin is someone who has not had sexual intercourse. One way that virginity is confirmed in a woman is whether her hymen is intact. The hymen is a weblike membrane that covers part of the entrance to the vagina. Often when it is stretched or broken (usually by penetration), bleeding occurs. This used to be the test for virgin brides. If there was not a spot of blood on the bedsheets the next morning, the husband was often shamed: He must not have married a virgin. We were told of one religion where it was a tradition that the marriage be consummated at the wedding reception, in a nearby room. In case there was no blood (which sometimes happens even when a hymen is present), a small container of chicken blood was made available so the couple could make the sheets "proper" for the wedding guests to see. And you thought *your* wedding night was special.

Anyway, sex isn't the only way for a woman to lose her hymen. Sometimes trauma, such as a blow or series of impacts to the body, can tear the hymen. Such trauma can occur if a woman rides a horse western style rather than sidesaddle.

The old wives were very concerned about their little girls being perceived as "experienced" before marriage, something that wasn't considered acceptable. There were even those who would try to "simulate" virginity. We won't go into detail, but a few of the methods included creative stitching and blood-soaked sponges.

Virginity will always have a special significance for some, which is why horseback riding is often discouraged for girls who don't know how to ride properly. As far as losing one's virginity on a horseback ride, we suppose it could be possible. Not comfortable, but possible.

CATS ARE PSYCHIC

*"Cats seem to go on the principle
that it never does any harm
to ask for what you want."*
JOSEPH WOOD KRUTCH, *TWELVE SEASONS,* "FEBRUARY"

Let's be honest here. We could come up with scientific evidence from Nobel Prize–winning researchers that says that there is no proof that cats possess some sort of psychic ability, but if we did there would be those who would scream bloody cat murder. In case you haven't noticed, cat lovers are a rather dedicated bunch. They can tell you stories about how their cat knows their moods and how the feline will do things that are almost human on purpose and how their little tabby predicted the big earthquake a few minutes before everyone else felt it.

Now let's be really honest. Cats are not psychic. (Now that it's been said, please don't scream. We like cats. We really do.) Cats, like dogs and other animals, rely on their senses for protection. Therefore, their senses of smell, touch, etc., are significantly more acute than those of humans. So when they show up suddenly in a room or react to something that you didn't hear, it's not ESP at work, it's their normal perceptions.

Consider the earthquake stories that you always hear. Pet owners swear that their animals go nuts *before* an earthquake strikes. They reason the cats must have known ahead of time that the earth was going to move. How else other than being psychic could they know? The earthquakes that humans feel are often preceded by smaller earthquakes. It is one of those smaller quakes, or the beginning of the larger quake that the cats react to. Because humans don't feel something, we assume it isn't there. Cats, though, with their acute sense of touch, react quite naturally to something they feel but that we may not.

This isn't to say that cats aren't special. Any cat lover will tell you that they are very affectionate animals. It is because they love their cats so much that they are more willing to attribute to them mystical or extrasensory qualities. It's often easier and more romantic to say that the cat did something amazing than to consider a more plausible explanation. Call us cynical, but the fact is that there have been no studies done that show that cats possess psychic abilities.

Cats have also been the subject of many other superstitions and misunderstandings. One is that their eyes glow in the dark. Cat's eyes are very reflective and do gleam when even the faintest light hits them, but they will not glow on their own. Another is that cats will always land on their feet. While cats are very agile and usually can right their bodies to land on their feet, there is no guarantee of this. There is also the belief that cats have nine lives. This began with the ancient Egyptians, who were enamored with cats and thought them to be holy. Nine was chosen because it is the product of three times three, three being the holiest of numbers. Unfortunately, although they might escape some situations due to their agility, cats only have one life.

Cats are loving, cute, friendly, and mysterious. But psychic they're not.

ONCE YOU FIND ROACHES IN YOUR HOUSE YOU CAN NEVER GET RID OF THEM

"As Gregor Samsa awoke one morning from uneasy dreams he found himself transformed in his bed into a gigantic insect."
FRANZ KAFKA, "THE METAMORPHOSIS"

If you've ever lived in a cheap apartment building or college dorm you probably know the disgusting and frustrating feeling of snapping on the lights in the kitchen in the middle of the night only to see roaches scurry for cover. And what's worse, it seems like not even nuclear war can kill them. (A researcher actually once proved that roaches are susceptible to about the same amount of radiation as humans, so, no, they *wouldn't* survive a nuclear war.)

Roaches are perceived as filthy insects, and we assume their presence indicates an unclean living space. The unfortunate truth is that anyone can get roaches. Just because your kitchen is spotless doesn't mean that you won't be visited. You could very easily bring one home in a shopping bag from the supermarket. Whether they stay or not is another matter. If you do keep a clean house your chances of having the creatures return is much less than if your floor were covered with yesterday's leftovers.

Roaches can seem invincible. However, there are insecticides and other substances that will kill them. Boric acid is one of the most effective and popular. (The bottom of a shoe is another.) The problem with some sprays or powders is that they simply can't get into the cracks and crevices where the roaches hide. So when you think you've covered the entire kitchen with powder and traps, the fact is that you probably haven't. And this adds to the roach's mystique of being invincible.

It's also believed that roaches have developed an immunity to some insecticides. This isn't true. The fact is that certain poisons do kill roaches. However, it's also true that you probably won't kill all of them at the same time because of the out-of-reach places in which many of them hide. It's when they return that people assume that the roaches have built up a resistance.

The hard truth is, there is no reason to think that we'll be rid of roaches anytime soon. There are just too many places for them to hide. And it's a sad fact that there is never just one roach. If you do see a roach in your kitchen, the best thing to do is put boric acid near any entrance or crack through which a roach might enter (be sure to keep kids and pets away, though). Then make certain you've put away any unfinished food, and keep sinks and counters free of crumbs and food particles. If roaches have nothing to eat, they won't come back. If they *do* keep coming back, call a professional exterminator. Despite what the old wives say, you *can* get rid of roaches. You just have to know where to find them.

BREAST MILK IS BETTER FOR BABIES THAN COW'S MILK

"Every luxury was lavished on you—atheism, breast-feeding, circumcision. I had to make my own way."
JOE ORTON, *LOOT*

Is breast milk better for babies? In a word, yes. Every female animal that becomes a mother produces milk to meet the particular needs of her babies. Cow milk has in it things baby cows need, goat milk has in it things baby goats need, and human breast milk has things in it that human babies need. Breast milk, then, is the result of a mother's natural function and babies naturally benefit from it.

Human breast milk has been shown to be just plain healthier for babies. Certain antibodies are passed to the baby by way of the breast milk. Breast milk cannot be contaminated like premade formulas. There are no cans or bottles involved. And babies are rarely if ever allergic to breast milk.

There are other reasons why many believe breast-feeding is best for a baby. One is that a baby's teeth and jaw will develop better if breast-fed. This is because the baby has to work a lot harder to get milk from a breast than from a bottle. In fact, a baby uses almost sixty times the amount of energy getting milk from a breast than it does getting the same amount of milk from a bottle. Babies are born with small pads of fat in their cheeks and lips to give them extra help in getting milk from a breast. These pads are gone by the time the child is a year old. Babies who are bottle-fed, and thus don't use the pads, sometime substitute their thumbs to satisfy the sucking need they're born with.

This isn't to say that breast-feeding is always better than bottle feeding or that breast-fed babies always turn out healthier. It is possible for a mother to pass along unhealthy substances, such as alcohol, drugs, or illnesses to their babies through their milk. Also, some people believe that babies given cow's milk grow to be bigger and have healthier bones since they get more calcium.

Ultimately, the choice is up to the mother. Most women find the psychological bonding that goes along with breast-feeding to be irreplaceable. And, from a logic standpoint, breast milk *is* better for a baby. So in this case, the old wives fed us the right stuff.

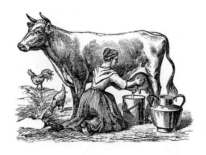

LEMON JUICE WILL GET RID OF FRECKLES

"Four be the things I'd been better without:
love, curiosity, freckles, and doubt."
DOROTHY PARKER, "INVENTORY"

What would Norman Rockwell have done without freckles? Not that his face was covered with them, but when he wanted to paint an All-American kid, he'd put a freckle-faced youngster behind a lemonade stand hawking his drink for a nickel. Freckles are cute. Freckles are a part of childhood. And now the old wives tell us that the kid can take the juice from some of his lemons, rub it on his face, and his freckles will fade away? There's something wrong with that.

Cultural image bashing aside, there actually is something wrong with using lemon juice to remove freckles. It doesn't work. A lot of redheads may be screaming right now, saying that as kids they used lemons and got rid of some freckles. (Before reading on, they might want to consult the chapter on redheads having terrible tempers.) In fact, books on home remedies often tell you to use lemon juice to remove freckles or age spots. Rubbing the juice into your skin twice a day works just as well as expensive fade creams, they say.

Freckles (the medical term is ephelides) cannot be removed by creams, lotions, or juices that merely bleach the skin. Why? Because the pigment-producing cells that cause freckles aren't on the surface of the skin. They're deeper. So when you fade freckles, you're not really removing them. If you go into the sun enough, the freckles will return in all their glory. There are some chemical peels that remove layers of skin to remove freckles, but this is only done in extreme cosmetic situations. There is also a technique called dermabrasion to remove freckles, and it's just as nasty as it sounds. Basically, dermabrasion shaves off layers of your skin. Obviously, this isn't recommended to take a few freckles off a kid's nose.

Once you have freckles, they don't go away. However, since exposure to sunlight is what causes freckles to appear, sunscreen may help. If freckles seem to fade as we grow older, it is only because we tend to be outside in the sunlight less than when we were kids. Increased exposure to the sun is also why we notice more freckles on our arms and face during the summer than in the winter.

So you might want to save your lemons for something other than rubbing them all over your freckles. Perhaps, in the spirit of Norman Rockwell, you could give them to a neighborhood kid and let him open up a lemonade stand. Unfortunately, with inflation, it's doubtful you'll be able to get a glass for a nickel anymore.

EAT PORK ONLY IN MONTHS WITH AN "R" IN THEM

"Pork. The other white meat."
ADVERTISEMENT FOR PORK

If this is true, then why have we been eating hot dogs during summer at the ballpark all these years? (Actually, who really knows what's in hot dogs anyway?)

Despite the fact that the old wives probably never took in a game, there is a little bit of common sense to this tale. But like most old-time, commonsense sayings, this one stayed around too long and probably scared more people than it helped.

One reason for this tale is the fear of trichinosis. Trichinosis is one of those parasitical diseases that your mother was so afraid of. This was responsible for millions of pork chops being cooked to their overdone death. Another reason was the state of refrigeration in the old days. Keeping things cold in the winter was no problem, but the summer was another matter. Pork needs to be refrigerated promptly and in the coldest part of the refrigerator, but in those days the coldest part of the refrigerator wasn't very cold. The term "ice box" was quite literal then. You didn't just plug in the fridge and store things in handy slide-out drawers. Instead, you relied on the ice man, who delivered large blocks of ice for you to use in an ice box as a way of preserving food. But as the ice melted, the temperature in the box—and everything stored in it—began to rise.

Also, in those days the quality of the meat sold in butcher shops wasn't always the best. We like to imagine an old-fashioned general store or butcher shop as having fresh fruit and meat, but the truth is that there were less rigorous standards back then.

These days, meat inspection is much stricter and refrigerators more effective, so the incidents of trichinosis are substantially fewer. In fact, the best way to avoid trichinosis is simply to cook pork thoroughly. It's recommended that you heat it until the internal temperature is at least 170 degrees Fahrenheit. But it's not really necessary to fry a pork chop until it can be used as a hockey puck.

So this wives' tale is not true. Eat all the pork you want, when you want. Have an extra hot dog at the game. You can pretend it has pork in it.

SIT-UPS WILL HELP GET RID OF LOVE HANDLES

··

"Being entirely honest with oneself is a good exercise."
SIGMUND FREUD, *ORIGINS OF PSYCHOANALYSIS*

What is this cruel trick that biology plays on men? When they reach their late twenties, they start to notice that tucking in their shirt is a little more difficult and their pants are just a little bit tighter. Then it happens. One day they look in the mirror and see a body they've never seen before but have feared all their lives. Oh my God, it's middle age!

Once men start to get middle-age spread, there is one universal piece of advice that has been around since, well, since the old wives started giving advice. Start doing sit-ups. Yes, the very exercise that people have hated since being forced to do them in junior high gym class.

The thought is that by doing sit-ups, you work on the middle of the body, right where the love handles are. Do a sit-up and you can feel your stomach muscles tighten. And since you're making your midsection do all the work, the fat in that area must be burning away, right?

Wrong. What people think they're doing is "spot reducing." In other words, they're trying to take off fat in a selected spot on their body, whether it's their stomach, their arms, or their behind. However, despite what infomercials for waist reduction products tell you, this is not possible. You can't remove fat from just one part of the body. You can tighten certain muscles, yes, but this is more for toning than it is for trimming weight.

The best way to lose weight and fat is to burn off more calories than you eat. In fact, you have to lose 3,500 calories to lose one pound. And there's no way to decide where that pound's going to come from. Sit-ups help burn fat, but it's much better to jog or do aerobic exercises. In fact, in a study at the University of Massachusetts, men who did almost 340 sit-ups a day for over twenty-seven days lost no significant fat in their midsections. There were still handles for love.

So this piece of advice from the old wives is just a tale. If you look in the mirror and happen to see your father's body looking back at you, you'll be much better off running around the block a few times and cutting down on your fat and caloric intake. Save your back and leave the sit-ups to the kids in junior high gym class.

A WOMAN CAN'T GET PREGNANT DURING HER PERIOD

....

"Only women bleed." ALICE COOPER, "ONLY WOMEN BLEED"

All good Catholics will recognize this one. Because the times a woman is fertile are determined by her menstrual cycle, if she can chart the days her cycle starts and stops, she can determine when she is most likely to become pregnant. Hence, she can also know when she is most likely *not* to become pregnant. This is known as the rhythm method of contraception.

In less modern times this was the preferred method of birth control. Back then, they didn't have reliable contraceptives so they had to rely on good old biology. These days birth control options include everything from pharmaceutical implants to fruit-flavored condoms.

Okay, great, but is the wives' tale true? Depends. Yes, there is a time during a woman's cycle when she probably won't get pregnant if she has unprotected sex. However, some women's cycles are longer than others and many women have irregular cycles, so the time they calculate as being safe is irregular also.

What this means, though, is that there are usually about five or six days during a woman's cycle where a couple can have sex and not worry about the woman getting pregnant. This leaves two problems: One is being absolutely sure that you figured the dates correctly. Two is having the discipline to limit yourselves to five or six specific days in a month. This makes the phrase "I'm in the mood for love" more a planned event than an actual mood.

So this old wives' tale is true to a point, but unless you do some pretty precise calculating, it might just be easier to drive down to your local pharmacy for a little insurance.

BREAST-FEEDING PREVENTS BREAST CANCER

....

*"Miss Manners' only objection about doing it (breast-feeding) discreetly is
the fear that babies don't breathe well under ladies' sweaters."*
MISS MANNERS, *MISS MANNERS' GUIDE TO EXCRUCIATINGLY CORRECT BEHAVIOR*

In a different chapter we talked about how good breast milk
and breast-feeding is for babies. In this chapter we thought
we'd give the mothers some good news.

According to some studies, this old wives' tale is true: breast-
feeding *does* help prevent breast cancer. Now, before we go
on we'd like to point out two things: One, there are some doctors and researchers who have seen no relationship between
breast-feeding and breast cancer. Some think there may be
more of a connection between pregnancy and cancer reduction. Two, nobody's really sure how breast-feeding even affects cancer.

Still, a recent study by the Centers for Disease Control found
that women who had children and breast-fed had significantly
less cancer. And it found that women who had more children
and breast-fed for even longer periods of time had even fewer
cases of breast cancer. And the protection seemed to last even
when the women got beyond their child-bearing years.

Another study at the Fred Hutchinson Cancer Research Center in Seattle, Washington, also found a big decrease in the
number of cases of breast cancer between women who breast-
fed and those who didn't. It also showed a lower incidence
in women who would normally have been in high-risk groups
but who breast-fed.

Again, these studies aren't conclusive and they never say
why breast-feeding seems to help prevent breast cancer, but
the old wives may have been on to something here. Tough
as it is to admit, it looks as though the medical community is
on their side. On this one, anyway.

WASHING YOUR HAIR IN RAINWATER MAKES IT CLEANER

"Then hadst thou had an excellent head of hair."
WILLIAM SHAKESPEARE, *TWELFTH NIGHT*

There are many flaxen-hair country girls who swear that this is true, and to be fair to flaxen-hair country girls everywhere there is some truth to this. (We wouldn't want them to get into a lather.) Rainwater has always had the reputation of being pure, sparkling, and clean.

If you think about it, all you need to wash your hair is soap and water. While it's obvious that different soaps have different ingredients, we may not realize that not all water is created, or delivered, equal. Water that comes from wells contains more minerals, for example, than rainwater. That's why it's known as "hard" water. Tiny as it is, the extra amount of calcium and magnesium in hard water can leave a residue on whatever is washed by it. These minerals, by the way, are also what cause that odor you notice coming from the faucet at Grandma's farm.

City water, or "soft" water, is treated, so many of the minerals are taken out. However, chemicals are added in the treatment process that make the water more acidic. Also, because this water travels through miles of pipe, particles of rust and whatever else may be in the pipe comes out of the showerhead along with the water.

Then there's rainwater. Compared to the other two possibilities, rainwater would seem like an obvious choice. Rain is clean, right? Actually, it depends. Sure, rain that falls in the most rural areas is relatively pure; in those places it *is* better to use rainwater because it has neither the minerals from wells, nor the chemicals from treatment plants. But, if you've ever seen New York or L.A. on a smoggy day, you can imagine what's in the rainwater in urban areas.

Storage is another thing to consider. If the rain comes out of the sky pure and clean, won't it be contaminated by whatever you store it in? Rain barrels are commonly used, but unless they're cleaned often, even rainwater takes on a smell that's not so heavenly.

So if you want the cleanest hair possible, grab your shampoo and head out to the farm and wait for a good low-pressure system. Two warnings: Don't expect the water to warm up after a few minutes, and check your local laws on public showering (or bring your own shower curtain).

SUNTAN OIL MAKES YOU TAN FASTER

"Hey, buddy, you're blocking my light."
THE GUY NEXT TO YOU ON THE BEACH

Blame it on Madison Avenue, blame it on California, blame it on George Hamilton, but part of the image of the young, tragically hip beach bunny or bum is a dark tan. Whether it's just a weekend tan or one that you've worked on for the whole summer (for some it's an art form), tans have come to be associated not only with good looks, but good health.

This being the case, suntan oil has become a big business. We used to slather on the Coppertone to get a tan more quickly. These days we know a lot more about the sun and what it can do to us. So, over the years, with the addition of ingredients that protect us from the sun's ultraviolet rays, "suntan oil" has become "sunscreen."

Sunscreens do just that—they screen out part of the sun. They absorb or reflect the sun's dangerous ultraviolet rays while allowing enough rays to penetrate and turn your skin darker. So suntan oil actually makes you tan more slowly.

We know now how dangerous the sun's rays are. There are a lot more cases of skin cancer being treated than ever before, and sunscreens are now strongly advised for those who are spending the day at the beach or lying in the sun. In fact, a tan is your skin's way of telling you that it's been injured. It produces the darker pigment to warn you and to help protect itself from the sun.

We hate to break the news to the tanning gods out there, but excessive tanning can age your skin really quickly. That tan that looks so great today can make your skin look and feel like leather when you reach your golden years. In fact, one way to prove it to yourself is to drop your pants. (Trust us.) Put the back of your hand up next to your backside. Compare the skin on both. Chances are the skin down below looks a lot smoother and younger than the skin on your hand. This is because your hand has been exposed to the sun all these years and your derriere has not.

And don't think that cloudy days are protection against sunburn. It's been found that up to 80 percent of ultraviolet rays penetrate clouds. In other words, you can get a sunburn on a day when you see no sun at all. The same is true for foggy days as well. You're not even safe from a sunburn if you have it "made in the shade." If you're beneath a shady tree, ultraviolet rays can still reach you by reflecting off the ground or nearby water. The bottom line is, if you're going outdoors, especially between 10:00 A.M. and 2:00 P.M., wear sunscreen for protection.

So this is a good wives' tale to ignore. Sunscreens help, but take our advice and don't even try to get a deep tan. A little sun feels good, but you don't want to grow old and wonder why your butt is the only part of you that looks your age.

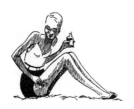

A DROWNING MAN COMES UP THREE TIMES
BEFORE STAYING UNDER

···

"Throw a lucky man into the sea and he will come up with a fish in his mouth." Arabic Proverb

Unfortunately, this is more wishful thinking than it is scientific fact. If you see a movie where someone is drowning you'll probably see them bobbing up and down, struggling to be saved. But, as the old wives sometimes refuse to believe, real life isn't like the movies.

In the case of drowning, there is no one way that people succumb. Some may go under and never come up, some may be stronger and be able to come up for air many times. The fact is that once people lose consciousness or can't manage to tread water anymore, they won't be able to surface. And it doesn't matter whether they've come up three times or not.

When someone is drowning, they put up a violent struggle, so it may look as though they return to the surface many times. They may, in fact, be able to surface three times, but there is nothing to suggest that this will be the same for everyone.

This is another example of our fascination with the number three. There are religious implications here having to do with the Holy Trinity. Three also is associated with death; many believe that famous people die in threes. How this number became associated with drowning isn't known.

There have been other tales dealing with drowning. It was once believed that people drowned not because they couldn't swim but because there was an evil spirit in the water. Sailors were so afraid of the water spirit that they would never say the word "drowning" while they were at sea. In fact, many years ago some sailors would not even try to rescue a man who was drowning. They were afraid that if the water spirit was denied a victim, someone would have to take his place. And who better than the man who saved the intended victim?

So this old wives' tale is not true at all. It's also not true that an evil spirit is in the lake, so if you see someone drowning, call the lifeguard as soon as you can. There's nothing magical about someone's drowning.

DREAMS PREDICT THE FUTURE

"For all life is a dream, and dreams themselves are only dreams."
PEDRO CALDERÓN DE LA BARCA, *LIFE IS A DREAM* (PLAY)

If you think we're able to answer this one to everyone's satisfaction, you're dreaming.

There are those who swear that they had a dream that later came true. Therefore, the dream predicted the future. There are also those who say that when this happens it's merely a coincidence or that the person didn't remember the dream the way it actually happened, thus making the memory of the dream fit what happened.

The bottom line is that no one can say for sure whether dreams predict the future or not. It's generally agreed that dreams reflect our thoughts and emotions. In the dream state we don't have any of the usual restraints that we normally have. We don't let logic get in the way, so anything can happen in a dream.

Some point to famous cases where a person's dream came true later on. One of the more well known is when Abe Lincoln dreamed that he saw his own casket in the White House, and when he asked someone who had been killed, the person in the dream responded that it was the president (Lincoln himself) and that he'd been assassinated by being shot. A few weeks later, Lincoln was assassinated in real life. Surely this must be proof.

Well, maybe not. Someone else might argue that after the Civil War, Lincoln was aware that there were many people in the country who didn't like him or his policies. So it must have crossed his mind a few times that there was the possibility of being assassinated. This being the case, his dream doesn't seem that unusual.

Scientists know some things about dreams and they're unclear on others. They know that most dreams take place when we're in deep sleep, know as rapid eye movement (REM) sleep. If you watch someone who's dreaming, you can actually see their eyes moving back and forth. It's also known that we dream every night. If you think you have a night without dreams, it's just that you don't remember them. Also, dreams can last anywhere from a few seconds to an hour.

However, what isn't so clear is what dreams mean. Everyone dreams about falling or being naked in front of a group of people or being unable to move. Whether this means the same thing for everyone is not so clear. Some go so far as to claim that certain objects in a dream can be interpreted the same for everyone. They'll tell you that dreaming of a carrot means that you'll get money soon. Dreaming of frogs means that you're happy with yourself and your friends. There are too many of these to mention, but, as the dream master himself, Sigmund Freud, once said: "Sometimes a cigar is just a cigar."

So there's no conclusive way to tell if this old wives' tale is true. Maybe it's just something they came up with in their sleep. But whatever you believe, before you go to bed tonight you might want to read the chapter on whether certain foods can give you nightmares. It's a fact that no one wants those dreams to come true.

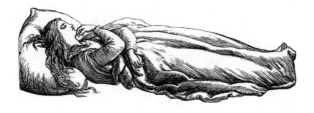

HOT TODDIES HELP CURE A COLD OR FLU

"There's no malice in me eye,
But I wish that they could cure the common cold.
That's all. Good-bye."
PAM AYERS, "OH, NO, I GOT A COLD"

You've got a cold. You're aching all over and it's almost impossible to breathe. The best thing to do is get some sleep, but the way you feel you think you'll never sleep again. To your rescue come the old wives.

For those of you who have never had one, a hot toddy can be made of many different ingredients. Usually it consists of hot water (the Hot), lemon, and either brandy or whiskey (the Toddy). Others use everything from herbal tea to honey or garlic.

Do they help? They can. First of all, drinking something hot should help loosen the congestion in your chest and nose. This won't clear you for good, but being able to breathe easier for a little while may help you sleep. The alcohol is also meant to help you sleep. Alcohol is a depressant, yes, but if you have too much it can make sleeping more difficult and it may interact negatively with the ingredients in some over-the-counter cold medicines.

The theory is that if you drink a hot toddy before going to bed, you'll be sleepier and its ingredients will make you sweat as you sleep, and keep your breathing passages open. While this may help with the symptoms of a cold, remember there's still no known cure.

So if your goal is to sleep a little better, then, yes, this old wives' tale is true. But if you think that drinking a hot toddy before bed is going to cure your cold, then you've been drinking too much toddy.

BEING OVERWEIGHT IS CAUSED BY OVEREATING

*"At a dinner party one should eat wisely but not too well, and talk well
but not too wisely."*
W. SOMERSET MAUGHAM, WRITER'S NOTEBOOK

This one seems like a no-brainer, right? It follows that if you eat the entire left side of the menu, you'll end up a pound or two over your normal weight.

Sure, this is true. Being overweight *can* be caused by overeating, but this isn't the only cause. The problem with some of the tales the old wives tell is that they may be partially true, but they ignore some important points.

Eating too much can make you weigh too much. But *what* you eat is also important. Recent studies have found that the amount of fat in your diet makes a difference in weight gain. In other words, someone whose diet consists of foods lower in fat can eat more than someone who eats a lot of hamburgers and chocolate shakes. In this case it's the content, not the amount, that contributes to weight problems.

And, of course, it's not as simple as watching how much and what you eat. You need to exercise as well. Doctors say that those calories that you eat need to be burned off. If they're not, they turn to fat cells that pad your waist and cling to your thighs. It's also recommended that you exercise right after eating (nothing too strenuous, though). This way, you'll double the number of calories you burn. So if you exercise enough you can compensate for eating more than you normally would.

As if that weren't enough, it also matters *when* you eat. The worst thing you can do is eat a large meal late in the day. It's then that the body burns off the fewest number of calories. In fact, one researcher found that we burn calories most efficiently during the first hour after we wake up. So breakfast should be the biggest meal we eat, lunch a little smaller, dinner not so big, and a midnight snack should only be in our dreams.

So while the old wives are right about this one, we'll only give them partial credit. After all, we can only swallow so much.

IT'S BAD LUCK FOR THE GROOM TO SEE THE BRIDE BEFORE THE WEDDING

"Can a maid forget her ornaments, or a bride her attire?"
JEREMIAH 2:32

Weddings and old wives' tales will be together forever (unlike many brides and grooms). Every family has their own traditions, and everyone knows of things that need to be done and shouldn't be done on the wedding day. It seems as though there's a superstition associated with nearly every aspect of a wedding, including how we dress, where we stand, and what we do on the honeymoon.

One of the most common wedding superstitions is that it is bad luck for the groom to see the bride on the day of the wedding before they meet at the altar. This tale has caused women to rush into churches and forced men to cover their eyes. The question is, has its violation been the cause of disastrous marriages?

With the divorce rate alarmingly high, there must be a good reason. There are many sociological explanations, but the fact that a man saw a woman in her wedding gown before the ceremony is not one of them. Simply put, there is no truth to this tale.

Where this superstition started, no one can say for sure. Some believe it's a spin-off of the tradition of a woman's wearing a veil during a wedding. The veil had a few meanings to it, one of which was the belief that the man shouldn't see his beloved until the moment he "possessed" her. The thought was that anything that was on display was not as valuable as something that was kept hidden. It was also a symbol of her submission to him. The veil was used in some cultures to protect the bride from evil spirits by hiding her until she was married. It's also thought that the veil derives from the wedding canopy, used in some Jewish and Catholic ceremonies. Again, the main point was to protect the bride and groom from anything evil that might prevent or harm the marriage. This is also the rationale behind the groom not seeing the bride before the ceremony.

However, this superstition is not always observed. In fact, in some cultures it was a tradition for the bride and groom to walk together to the church along with their wedding party. So not only did he see her before the wedding, they would actually spend some time together. And we'd be willing to bet that the rate of failed marriages was a lot less back then than it is now.

There are many other traditions that go along with weddings and there are just as many theories about how those traditions began. Following these customs makes the event more fun for some and makes others more paranoid. But there is no reason to believe that bad luck will result if the groom sees the bride. Now it may become bad luck if they both believed in it and it happened. But, superstitions aside, there are much more important (and real) factors that contribute to a successful marriage. After all, we're sure that many marriages that started with the groom not seeing the bride ended and many marriages that started with the groom seeing the bride worked out well.

And so, do we believe that this old wives' tale might be fun to observe but is ridiculous to believe, from this day forward?

We do.

PRESS A HALF-DOLLAR AGAINST A WOUND TO STOP THE BLEEDING

"He jests at scars, that never felt a wound."
WILLIAM SHAKESPEARE, *ROMEO AND JULIET*

As far back as the days of alchemists, metallic objects have been believed to have healing powers. Certain metals could cure diseases or ward off spirits, they knew.

It was once believed that gold had a connection to the human heart. The element was actually ingested (yes, swallowed) to help with heart ailments. Silver was more of a thinking man's metal. It was a sure cure for poor memories. Even a metal as plain as iron had its uses. In the old days, people kept an iron horseshoe near their front door to ward off witches and evil spirits. They would even wear iron jewelry to protect their bodies from these spirits.

For centuries, then, people have used metals to cure and prevent afflictions. Half-dollars were introduced in America in the mid-1800s, when there was still a fascination with the healing power of metals. In fact, up until 1964 half-dollars were 90 percent silver. So it's not hard to see how they would be associated with such curing power.

But what's this fifty-cent wives' tale worth? Well, there is a grain of truth here. Doctors tell us that the best way to stop bleeding is to apply direct pressure to the wound. This helps the blood clot, which stops the bleeding and allows the skin to begin healing. This is the purpose of bandages, that and to keep the wound safe from dirt and infection.

Pressing a half-dollar to a wound would, in fact, help stop the bleeding because it would clog the opening through which the blood is flowing. However, half-dollars aren't the cleanest or most sanitary of objects to place against an open wound. So while the bleeding might stop, the risk of infection may increase, depending on where the half-dollar's been.

Therefore, unless you want to go to the trouble of boiling your coins to remove the germs, it might just be easier to take them to the pharmacy and buy a small box of bandages.

NICE GUYS FINISH LAST

....

"Walker. Cooper. Mize. Marshall. Kerr. Gordon. Thomson. Take a look at them. All nice guys. They'll finish last. Nice guys. Finish last." LEO DUROCHER DESCRIBING HIS TEAM

This tale, of course, started with that famous old wife Leo Durocher. Leo managed the Brooklyn Dodgers and the Chicago Cubs for many years, and if you know anything about baseball you know that the Cubs know what it takes to finish last. Durocher saw his team as pleasant enough fellows, but as far as winning went, there was nothing nice about them.

Like many famous quotes, this one changed a bit over the years into a shorter, more convenient piece of wisdom. But, baseball aside, do nice guys always finish last? Is it part of their disposition that someone will always push them around and claim the prize instead? Will the nice guy always let him get away with it? It may seem that way, but just because you're nice doesn't mean you'll always (or ever) finish last.

The saying today is applied to business situations where it's thought that aggressiveness equals success. If you are ruthless and have no morals, then it is easy to succeed. Meanwhile, the person who plays by the rules will always be left behind. This is a generalization and a poor one at that.

Also coming into play here is the image we all have of the lovable loser, that person who always finds a way to screw up and in the end lose the girl or not get the promotion. This is a standard character in most comedies. He may be a loser, but he's nice and we like him anyway.

Do nice guys always finish last? No. Do rotten guys always win. Of course not. So while this saying may give comfort to people who lose at something, it's certainly not a given that it was kindness that made them lose. After all, even some not-so-nice people have played for the Cubs over the years.

FAMOUS PEOPLE DIE IN THREES

"In the future, everyone will be world-famous for fifteen minutes."
ANDY WARHOL

Let's say that you're watching television and you hear that a famous actor died. Then a few days later it's reported that a former world leader passed away. You then know for sure that someone else famous is going to die soon. Why? Because it always happens in threes. Always.

At least that's what the old wives would have us think. And if you think about it, we can't really prove that they're wrong on this one. But then again, they can't really prove that they're right. Does this sound confusing? Let us explain.

People die all the time; this is an unfortunate fact of life. And despite what their press agents would have us think, famous folks are human, too. And there has never been a proven pattern to the number of people dying. Sure, the number will fluctuate because of war or demographics or natural disasters, but there has never been a steady pattern established in terms of people dying in groups.

Then why does it seem like famous people die in threes? There's a very good explanation for this. It's because we look for it in threes. Think about it. If a famous person dies, then another one is certain to die at some point, and another at a certain point beyond that. So, technically, yes, they die in threes, but if that's the case then everyone dies in threes if we choose to look at it that way. After all, no one said if there is a certain time limit within which they have to die. Therefore, if one celebrity dies in January, a second celebrity dies in mid-January, and a third celebrity dies in mid-February, then they died in a group of three. And this also would have been true if the third celebrity had died a month later. See how it works?

Again, this goes back to our fascination with the number three. Whether it has religious significance or superstitious value, we always tend to put things in threes. (Wouldn't it be convenient if there were three old wives who started all this?)

It's also been said that disasters happen in threes. If there is a plane crash and an earthquake within a relatively short period of time, everyone expects another type of disaster to occur.

What a lot of people never notice is that they also happen in twos or fours. If three celebrities die close together or if three disasters happen within a certain time, we take notice. But if they don't, we don't draw as much attention to it. So in a way we're convincing ourselves that these things *do* happen in threes.

The bottom line is that this old wives' tale isn't true, no matter whether you hear it once or whether you hear it three times.

YOU CAN'T TAN THROUGH A WINDOW

*"Give me the splendid silent sun
with all its beams full-dazzling."*
WALT WHITMAN, "GIVE ME THE SPLENDID SILENT SUN"

It's a nice day so you go out for a long drive in the car. You roll down the window and put your arm out while you drive. When you get to where you were going, you notice that the arm that was resting in the open window has a red, painful sunburn and the arm that was inside the car is perfectly fine, although it was in the sun that came through the window. You wonder why. Naturally, the old wives have an answer for you. You can't get a tan from sunlight that comes through window glass.

While most people don't think twice about sitting in the sunlight coming through a window in their house, this question usually arises during long car trips. If you've ever driven for hours and hours in the sun and wanted to avoid a sunburn on your face, you would remember being told by the backseat old wives to close the window so the glass would stop the sun's rays from burning you.

The old wives were right about this one, too. To shed a little light on the subject without getting too technical, suntans and sunburns are caused by ultraviolet rays. If you spend a lot of time outdoors, you're told to wear sunscreen to block out these rays and protect your skin. (See the chapter on suntan oil.) Being in direct sunlight for even a short time can be harmful to the skin. And it's between the hours of 10:00 A.M. and 2:00 P.M. that you have to be extra careful, when the sun is the most direct and the ultraviolet rays the strongest.

But what if you're by the window or in your car during these hours and the sun is shining? Don't worry. Most of the harmful rays can't get through windows because of the density of the glass. Even though glass is clear, the particles that make up glass block certain wavelengths of light from passing through. Yes, some of the rays that cause your skin to burn will get through, but not enough to burn you very quickly. If you were to spend an entire day in the sun behind a window or windshield, you might get a slight tan, but not a burn. However, you can burn in only a few hours of direct sunlight. This shows just how much glass windows do cut down on the ultraviolet rays.

So the next time you plan a long trip in the car and you don't want to end up with one arm raw and the other well done, roll up the windows and keep both hands on the wheel.

IF YOU URINATE ON THE THIRD RAIL OF THE SUBWAY TRACKS, YOU'LL BE ELECTROCUTED

"Awaiting the sensation of a short, sharp shock."
GILBERT AND SULLIVAN, *PATIENCE*

Who knew the old wives rode the subway? They've been warning us for years that if we go down into a subway tunnel and urinate on the tracks, we could kill ourselves—and not from embarrassment. There are three rails that make up subway tracks, and the third rail is what's known as a "hot" rail. The third rail is like an exposed wire, except that it has over six hundred volts running through it. So, if you were to take a "comfort break" directly onto that third rail, you would be exposing yourself to danger because water is a very good conductor of electricity. The rationale is that once the water hit the rail, the electricity would travel up through the stream, into your body, and kill you.

In theory, this would be true. Water *is* a good conductor of electricity and if a steady stream of "water" passed between you and a source of electricity, it would be possible for you to get shocked. If you've ever been shocked by even low-voltage electricity, you know what happens. The jolt from the shock pushes you away from the source of the electricity. If you were being shocked because of a stream of water coming out of you, and you were to move even a little bit, then your "aim" would be off and the connection would be broken. Therefore, it would be difficult to maintain the connection long enough for this to be deadly. Actually, though, there are only a small number of cases where this has happened. Figuring the number of people who have probably tried this we can assume that not everyone who does this gets the shock of their lives.

Technically, though, the old subway wives are right about this one. So if you find yourself in a subway and facing a long line at the public restroom, we suggest standing in line just a bit longer. While the chances of the "third rail shock" killing you during urination aren't as high as some might think, we're sure that no one really wants to see you try.

YOU CAN GET AIDS OR HERPES IN A HOT TUB

"Noble deeds and hot baths are the best cures for depression."
DODIE SMITH, *I CAPTURE THE CASTLE*

Picture yourself at a hip Malibu party, and all the beautiful people decide to take their expensive drinks and jump into the hot tub for a little social soaking. Everyone's discussing their latest movie deal when suddenly they hear, "Mind if we join you?" And standing there in their bikinis are the old wives. End of party.

But before they would ever go into a hot tub, the old wives would want the water drained and the tub scrubbed because they always told us that we can get AIDS or herpes from being in water that was shared with people who have those diseases. They figure that the viruses that cause these diseases would breed even more in such a warm, damp environment.

It's commonly believed that HIV, the AIDS virus, doesn't survive outside the body. The only way it can be spread is through direct transmission of bodily fluids from one person to another or through infected blood. The herpes virus cannot survive in temperatures much warmer than the human body, so it cannot be transmitted through warm water. So, there's very little chance of ever being infected with either of these viruses solely by sharing a hot tub.

There have been reports, though, of the herpes virus being able to survive outside the human body and being transferred from one person to another on, say, the seat outside a hot tub. Again, it depends on the temperature of the seat.

This doesn't mean that you can't pick up other kinds of infections from a jacuzzi or a hot tub. If the water you're sitting in is dirty enough, there is a chance you could get sick. Hot tub owners usually don't add chemicals like chlorine to their hot tubs the way they do their swimming pools. This is because the water in swimming pools is usually left standing longer and therefore needs to be treated. Hot tubs are much smaller, so changing the water and disinfecting the tub aren't such big deals.

So if someone invites you into a hot tub, don't worry about getting either AIDS or herpes from the water. You might, however, want to consult the chapter on losing your love handles before exposing yourself to the beautiful people.

YOU CAN'T PHOTOGRAPH INTO THE SUN

"Sunshine on the water looks so lovely."
JOHN DENVER, "SUNSHINE ON MY SHOULDERS"

There you are at a wedding with everyone gathered around the bride and groom outside the church. You're all set to take some pictures when you hear the annoying voice of the old wives telling the bride not to stand where she is because the sun is behind her. None of your pictures will come out, they tell you, because it's impossible to take a picture with the sun behind the subject. It'll make them either overexposed or make the bride and groom merely a dark blur. The rule is: "You can't take a picture with the sun in front of you," they say.

While photography has become relatively easy (especially

with instant cameras), there are still some common misconceptions about it. Photographing into the sun is one of them. We decided to consult an expert on this one. We talked to professional cinematographer Bruce Dorfman and posed this wives' tale to him. "It's obviously not true," he said. Of course, if you just pointed a camera directly into the sun you could have a tough time. To get around the problem, he suggests that you simply block the sun with the person being photographed or with a house or a tree. Or you can simply shade the sun with your hand to control the amount of light the camera lets in through its opening, or aperture. This is also know as the f-stop. F-stops range from f2 to about f16; the higher the number the smaller the opening. Smaller openings are used with more light.

Dorfman added that there are artistic preferences to consider as well. "Front lighting is the most boring way to shoot things," he said. "It makes the picture look two-dimensional. There are no shadows. It's best to use side or back lighting. I would never, for instance, use only front lighting for a movie unless I was trying to achieve a flatter look." So in some cases you might want to have the sun in front of you to give the subject some depth. You might also want to create a silhouette effect. You'd probably achieve this with most automatic cameras if the sun were in front of you.

Dorfman went on to say that professional wedding photographers use a flash to counteract the sun. While the sun is behind the bride adding a nice glow surrounding her hair, the flash fills in the light on her face and make her features more visible (something most brides want in their wedding pictures). You can see what different lighting angles can do for a photo subject simply by having a person hold a light directly above their face, below it, behind their head, and to either side. The results can make a person look mysterious, evil, or even angelic, depending on how he is lit.

So this old photographers' wives' tale isn't true. Those who know photography use the light to their advantage. "It's a matter of controlling where the light comes from," said cinematographer Dorfman. "You don't have to necessarily work with what nature gives you."

Nor do you have to listen to the advice the old wives give you.

SETTING OUT PLASTIC JUGS FULL OF WATER WILL STOP DOGS FROM SOILING YOUR LAWN

"That indefatigable and unsavory engine of pollution, the dog."
JOHN SPARROW, LETTER TO THE *NEW YORK TIMES*

Anyone with a front lawn or a backyard has wondered about how to keep the neighborhood dogs from paying a visit and leaving a special gift. Some towns have laws requiring dog owners to follow their hounds with scoopers and plastic bags, but those same towns also have laws against jaywalking and look how much good that does.

The only way to avoid having a dog leave his business on your lawn is to stand guard twenty-four hours a day. Since this doesn't work into most people's schedules, someone figured the next best thing would be to develop something to scare away the pups or at least to discourage them from using their lawn as a rest stop. It would be sort of a dog-scarecrow, we guess.

No one knows for sure when, but at least as far back as the 1970s someone came up with the unique idea that if you took plastic gallon jugs, cut off their tops, filled them halfway with water, and placed them along the borders of your lawn, dogs would be spooked into not entering your property. For a while, this was a common sight, and even today you can still see few grassy areas lined with plastic jugs. This is an international wives' tale, for in New Zealand, home owners have been known to put clear bottles of water on their lawns for the same purpose.

So does this work? The real question should be, *how* does it work? Some say that the dogs don't know what the jugs are, and this stops them. There is a certain amount of familiarity and habit in dogs' restroom routines that having the jugs there disrupts. Others say that if you put a foul-smelling substance, such as ammonia, in the water, the smell will keep the dogs away.

Well, we're sorry to say that this is an old dogs' tale. There is no real reason for this to work. Sure, dogs might initially be frightened by the odd sight of decapitated milk cartons, but they'd eventually adjust and go back to business as usual. And the smell of the ammonia would probably keep them away, but then you'd have to ask yourself if it's worth it having a permanent smell on your property.

Look at it this way. You're trying to stop dogs from making your lawn look ugly. But what you're doing to accomplish this makes the lawn look a little ridiculous, too. The best thing to do is ask your neighbors to clean up after their pets. Or build a fence.

We hate to say it, but the old wives are just wrong on this one, doggoned.

GRIZZLY BEARS CAN BE ATTRACTED BY MENSTRUATING WOMEN

"Exit, pursued by a bear." WILLIAM SHAKESPEARE, *THE WINTER'S TALE*

We never knew that the old wives liked the outdoors, but in this case we're glad they do. Anyone who's ever taken a camping trip to the back country where bears live will tell you that it's a common piece of advice that women who are having their periods should not be out in the woods. This is because, they say, bears will be attracted to the smell of blood and possibly attack.

So is this good advice? Yes, it is. The grizzly, or Ursus arctos horribilis as it's known in scientific circles, has pretty bad eyesight. However, his sense of smell is quite acute. Bears are known to be able to smell humans over great distances. And because they are carnivores (meat eaters) one of the scents they notice most is the smell of blood. This can be any blood, however. There is nothing special about menstrual blood that attracts bears, just that it is blood. And since this will get the bears' attention, women are advised to stay out of the woods during their periods.

The best way to deal with grizzly bears is to avoid them. They are huge animals, the largest carnivores in North America. When they're on their hind legs they can stand as tall as eight feet. They can weigh up to a quarter of a ton. But just because they're big doesn't mean they're not fast. A bear can run faster than a human. According to the book *Night of the Grizzlies,* a bear can run three hundred yards in about twenty seconds. Humans are considered quite fast if they can run two hundred yards in that same twenty seconds. This is one reason why you don't want to give the bear any reason to come sniffing around your campsite. And don't think the nearest tree will save you. Despite what you may have heard, grizzly bears *can* climb trees.

So if you love the great outdoors, be sure to take the proper precautions. And if you're going to be in bear country, remember that bears can smell blood from great distances. One of the precautions you should take is to schedule your trip at a time when no one in your party will be menstruating. As if that time of the month weren't bad enough, you don't want to make it worse.

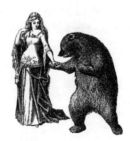

IF YOU PUT YOUR TONGUE ON THE HANDLE OF A WATER PUMP IN WINTER YOU'LL STICK TO IT UNTIL SPRING

....

"What freezings have I felt, what dark days seen!"
WILLIAM SHAKESPEARE, "SONNET 97"

This one may sound familiar to those readers who grew up on a farm. For those too young or too urban to know what we're talking about, before the development of electric water pumps, people used to get their water from underground wells by pumping the handle of a mechanical water pump that was usually outdoors. As a warning, older people would tell the younguns not to put their tongues on the pump's metal handle in winter or else they'd be stuck there until spring. This warning has been given in various forms throughout the years. Some of you may have heard a version where you weren't supposed to stick your tongue on a flagpole in winter. One friend even said he was told as a child to keep his tongue off of metal fences surrounding vacant lots (this is the city version).

The common ingredients in all these pieces of advice are cold, metal, and tongues. Probably the first question that comes to mind is why anyone would ever *want* to put his or her tongue on a water pump, a flagpole, or a fence regardless of the season. One answer is that this warning is usually directed toward young children, who will put anything in their mouths.

The explanation is that when your tongue makes contact with the cold metal, the moisture on the surface of the tongue freezes, thus keeping you in that position until things warm up—or, according to the tale, until spring thawed everything.

Basically, this is true. If a moist tongue is placed in contact with something cold enough to freeze water, then it will stick to it. And it'll stay there until the temperature of the surface of the object is raised. Sure, you could try to pull the tongue away, but that could be rather painful if the bond is strong enough between the tongue and the metal. Usually, warm water is enough to melt the connection and send the person on his way.

So the basic principle here is true. You probably wouldn't have to wait until spring, assuming there were some mildly intelligent people around. Of course, the best way to avoid looking ridiculous is to listen to the old wives and keep your tongue to yourself during winter.

HANG A SILVER SPOON IN CHAMPAGNE TO KEEP IT CARBONATED

"Life is mostly froth and bubble. . . ."
Adam Lindsay Gordon, "Ye Wearie Wayfarer"

You've counted down the New Year. You've kissed everyone at midnight. You've eaten all you can eat and drunk all you can drink. All that remains to take care of are the people who won't leave and the half-finished bottles of champagne. You look around for a reusable stopper since champagne corks expand so much that you can never get them back in the bottle. There are none. Since you don't want to drink flat champagne tomorrow, you figure you'll just pour it out since there's no way to preserve the carbonation. Suddenly a familiar voice comes from beneath the lampshade: "Wait! Don't pour it out yet!"

How the old wives got invited to your party we'll never know, but they go on to tell you that the best way to keep the bubble in your bubbly it to take a silver spoon and insert the handle into the bottle's opening. Let it hang there while the bottle is kept in the refrigerator, and the next day the fizz will still be fizzing. It's true, they say, and before passing out the old wives add that it'll save you money because you won't have to pour all that expensive liquid down the drain.

Does this really work? We thought we'd ask some experts. Unfortunately, a random sampling of some of the better establishments in Los Angeles turned up some not-so-conclusive results. Some winery workers said yes, it's supposed to work, and some said no, the spoon has no effect.

To our rescue came the Internet. On it we found a recent study where a group of researchers at the University of California at Berkeley decided to test the silver spoon theory. They took several bottles of champagne, opened them all, drank from them, and left some in each. They then left some bottles unprotected, put silver spoons in some and stainless steel spoons in others, and left them all in the fridge overnight. In the morning, they found that the silver spoon had no effect whatsoever. Obviously, putting a plastic stopper on the bottle would save the carbonation. But the champagne "protected" by the silver spoon went flat just as quickly as the unprotected champagne.

What may lead people to believe that a silver spoon helps is that some champagne keeps its carbonation in an open bottle for a few days anyway, with nothing sealing it. So if you put a spoon in it the fizz stays anyway. People may think that it's the spoon working its magic, but all along it's the champagne itself.

There is another, more plausible use for a spoon when handling champagne. If after you pop the cork from the bottle the champagne foams and starts to spill, you can stick a spoon handle into the bottle and hold the bottle at a forty-five-degree angle. This should contain the foam.

The bottom line, though, is that a spoon handle will not keep champagne carbonated. This old wives' tale is not true. So save your silver spoons for more important things, like eating. And if you serve champagne with dinner, either buy a plastic stopper or invite some Berkeley researchers to join you. Then you won't have to worry about leftovers.

CRACKING YOUR KNUCKLES WILL GIVE YOU ARTHRITIS

···

"Snap. Crackle. Pop." Rice Krispies

Is there anything in life more annoying than someone who constantly cracks their knuckles? And it's not just the sound it makes, but how much they love to torment you with it. And it's not only that. People also have different styles of cracking. They pull their fingers, bend their arms, and twist their wrists. It becomes habit-forming, they tell you. It feels good.

To get them to stop, their mothers would warn them that cracking their knuckles would lead to arthritis. They would end up with swollen, deformed hands that would make the Wicked Witch of the West look like a hand model.

Does knuckle cracking lead to arthritis? We consulted orthopedic surgeon Dr. Robert Bielski for this one. He explained it in precise medical detail, and when we told him we didn't understand a word he'd said, he put it in layman's terms.

He started by describing what actually happens when you crack your knuckles. What you're doing is hyperextending the joints in the fingers very rapidly. There is fluid in the joints and if it's forced from one section to another very quickly, there is a resulting cracking sound. He said the actual cause of the sound is really still just a theory.

Anyway, surrounding these joints are ligaments. And when you hyperextend the joints, you stretch these ligaments beyond their normal capacity. And when they stretch out, the fingers don't articulate normally. Dr. Bielski said that this can lead to degenerative changes and chronic deformity. In other words, your hand will take on shapes you never thought possible. In the old days, this was thought to be the result of arthritis. In reality, it's the ligaments that lead to the deformity.

Arthritis is a completely different problem with different treatments. You won't get arthritis with this habit, but your hands could suffer. The best way to stop the effects of knuckle cracking is simply to stop cracking your knuckles.

So while this old wives' tale isn't true, it is true that cracking your knuckles now can lead to problems for your hands later. Once again, your mother was right (sort of).

HITTING YOUR WRIST WITH A BIBLE WILL MAKE BUMPS GO AWAY

"From ghoulies and ghosties and long-leggety beasties
And things that go bump in the night, Good Lord, deliver us!"
CORNISH PRAYER

This is one from the midwestern old wives. According to this tale, people get what are called Bible Bumps. These are small, rubbery nodules that appear under the skin on the back of the hand or wrist or on the front side of the wrist where you take a person's pulse. When you see these bumps you're supposed to get rid of them by taking a Bible and whacking them with it. The bumps will then be gone.

We consulted a physician who said that without question this is actually true. Hitting those bumps with a Bible really does remove them. But, he went on to say, "It has nothing to do with the good word."

Bible Bumps are, in medical terms, small ganglions found under the skin. They are herniations of material that emanates from the lining of the wrist. The ganglion is a small pouch filled with gelatinous fluid. So when you take a Bible and smack it, the pouch bursts. The fluid then goes into the surrounding tissue, and the bump goes away. (It's unknown why it happens in the first place, but the lining of joints can produce this fluid as a natural occurrence.)

But it doesn't matter whether it's a Bible you use to break the sac or the local phone book. It's the force of the blow, not the content of the book, that makes the pouch rupture. This is not a treatment that lasts forever, though. The tear in the sac heals, it fills back up with the fluid, and then the bump is back. If you find that you have these bumps, you'll notice that they come and go a lot. Usually the bump shrinks in size spontaneously even without giving it a good smacking with the good book.

Of course, if you see any type of abnormal growth anywhere on your body you should see your doctor immediately. But if he tells you that it's simply a Bible Bump, you'll know what to do.

CABBAGE CAN REDUCE BREAST SWELLING

"Cauliflower is nothing but cabbage with a college education."
MARK TWAIN, *THE TRAGEDY OF PUDD'NHEAD WILSON*

Now when most people hear that cabbage can help with the engorged breasts of lactating women, they probably assume that the suggestion has to do with adding some cabbage to her diet. No, we actually mean sticking a piece of cabbage inside the woman's bra and keeping the cabbage next to her breast. And guess what? It's true. Talk about a wonder bra . . .

This is one of those American folk remedies that sounds weird but actually has a basic, sound, scientific reason for being effective. According to the *Jerusalem Post,* a study was done recently at Rambam Hospital. They took thirty women who had recently had babies. All complained of breasts that were too swollen due to lactation. Half of them were given green cabbage leaves to put in their bras (the red kind won't work). The other half used the usual methods of treating swelled breasts, including massage and warm compresses. The results of the study were that the normal methods didn't always work, but the women who used the cabbage said that their swelling went down considerably. Every one of them. The cabbage worked.

But do you have to have cabbage next to you all day? No, they said that putting the cabbage leaves in their bras for thirty minutes three times a day did the trick. Further, it was found that lactation stopped altogether if the cabbage was used more frequently.

The reason this works so well is that green cabbage is high in sulfa compounds. When these are absorbed into the skin (which they would be by wearing them inside a bra) they tend to constrict the passages through which the breast milk flows. This leads to less swelling. Simple.

So as odd as it may sound, this old wives' tale is true. And the next time you see a new mother with a piece of cabbage sticking out of her blouse, you'll know it's not there for support.

YOU CAN BREAK A GLASS BY SINGING A CERTAIN NOTE

"I do not mind what language an opera is sung in so long as it is a language I don't understand." SIR EDWARD APPLETON, ARTICLE IN *OBSERVER*

Remember those television commercials where they promoted a certain brand of audio tape by showing a famous singer shatter a wineglass simply by singing? Do you also remember that after you saw that demonstration you went into the kitchen, got out a cheap drinking glass, and started singing your lungs out to no avail? So was it you or were they faking it? Can you really shatter a glass by singing loudly?

Well, yes, in a way. But how loudly you sing is only part of it. What the whole thing boils down to is something called forced oscillation resonance. Okay, we'll explain it in English. A wineglass has a certain rate at which it vibrates. If you tap it, it makes a ringing noise. This is the sound of the glass vibrating. If you've ever seen anyone playing a series of glasses filled with varying levels of water, this is how they get the different "notes." The water makes the glasses vibrate at different rates and, thus, they make different sounds.

What a singer has to do in order to break a glass with his or her voice is duplicate the vibration rate of that glass. The note they sing with their voice has to make the glass vibrate at the exact same frequency as it would naturally. And if the note is loud enough and sustained long enough to get the glass really vibrating, then it will break. They say that only good singers can do this because it requires perfect pitch and the ability to sustain the note for a long enough time at a high enough volume. It's still debated whether a human can reach that volume without assistance. In the television commercial where the glass is shattered, the singer's voice is amplified by a speaker. Some form of amplification is usually needed.

The quality of the glass is also significant. It's better to use crystal since it has a high lead content and vibrates truer. A cheaper glass would be unevenly made and vibrate unevenly as well.

So this one is true. Technically, the human voice can shatter glass by hitting a certain note. And if you decide that you'd like to amaze your friends and break all your fine crystal, we might suggest a few singing lessons and good set of speakers.

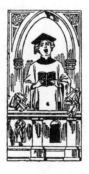

BATS WILL FLY INTO YOUR HAIR AND LAY EGGS IN IT

··

"Twinkle, twinkle little bat!
How I wonder what you're at!
Up above the world you fly,
Like a teatray in the sky."
LEWIS CARROLL, *ALICE'S ADVENTURES IN WONDERLAND*

If you grew up seeing bats flying around at dusk you can understand why some people think that bats might get into someone's hair. They don't fly in a straight path, and to humans their flight pattern is haphazard at best.

First, let's get one point out of the way. Bats don't want to fly into your hair. They have no reason to attack humans unless they are provoked or handled. If you leave a bat alone, he'll return the favor. But, people also fear bats because they've seen movies that show bats biting people. However, this doesn't happen very often in real life. There is also the fear that bats can spread rabies. Bats are actually one of the few creatures that can survive rabies. However, this danger is usually exaggerated. In fact, over the past thirty years there have only been ten deaths in the United States due to bites from rabid bats.

In other words, bats are not out to get you. It's also very unlikely that a bat would accidentally fly into your hair (even if you have the Don King look). Bats are quite good navigators and can fly in the dark very well. Around 1941, scientists discovered that bats actually fly by ear, using their ability to hear supersonic sounds to guide them. In fact, the bat is the only mammal capable of true flight.

Still, people fear the worst from this animal. Bats have always had an evil, mystical quality to them. In the Middle Ages, they were thought to be in league with the devil and with witches, able to transform themselves into humans or other species at will. Bram Stoker's *Dracula* exemplified this characterization to great dramatic effect, frightening generations of readers and moviegoers alike. Most cartoons featuring a wizard conjuring up a magic potion include bat wings as one of the ingredients. It was once believed that if a person smeared bat's blood on their face they could see better in the dark. Eating parts of the bat specially cooked was once a cure for asthma.

But what about bats flying into people's hair? In France, they once believed that if a bat were to fly into a woman's hair, she would have bad luck romantically or perhaps die within a year. There's no real explanation for *why* this would occur, but, as with most old wives' tales and superstitions, there doesn't have to be a clear reason for people to believe in something.

In reality, bats are actually beneficial to humans. They eat insects that are pests to humans, especially mosquitos. Sure, they can be annoying. Bats can live in your attic and they can make quite a squeaking noise. They can also leave droppings all over. However, bat droppings, or guano, is one of the best fertilizers. In fact, groups often organize expeditions to caves to collect guano.

If you see bats flying around, there's no need to get out the hats and hair nets. Chances are the bats won't be the least bit interested in flying into your hair. And if they do, they certainly won't stay in long enough to lay their eggs. This is, of course, because bats are mammals and don't lay eggs. Bats usually only give birth once a year and normally have just one baby at a time.

So don't worry about bats. Like most misunderstood animals, if you leave them alone they'll leave you alone.

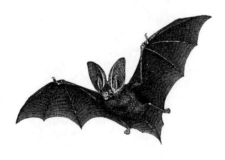

DON'T LOOK AT AN ECLIPSE OR YOU'LL GO BLIND

···

"My eyes were blind with stars and still I stared into the sky."
RALPH HODGSON, "THE SONG OF HONOUR"

R emember when you were in school and your science teacher announced that there was going to be an eclipse in the near future? Your project was always to construct one of those cardboard view-boxes. You could stand with your back to the sun holding the box on your shoulder, and the light from the sun was supposed to cast a shadow through a pinhole that would show the progress of the eclipse. It was supposed to. We don't know about you, but those boxes never worked for us.

A solar eclipse, simply put, is when the moon travels between the earth and the sun. Depending on the orbit of both bodies, an eclipse can be partial or total. Total eclipses, which cause a brief period of darkness, are fairly rare. Usually, eclipses only partially block the sun.

Okay, but what about looking at one? Do we have to rely on National Geographic specials or those cardboard boxes to see what's going on up there? Let's put it this way: If you were to take this old wives' tale literally, then, no, it's not true. Looking at a *total* eclipse during the few minutes when the moon completely blocks the sun will not make you go blind. What *can* hurt your eyes is looking at a partial eclipse or directly at the sun itself.

Think back to when you were a kid. Remember taking a magnifying glass and holding it in the sunlight just right? You could focus the light and burn a leaf or piece of paper in just a few seconds. Well, consider that the human eye works somewhat like a magnifying glass; it focuses the available light onto the retina, a fairly delicate piece of equipment. So looking directly at the sun for even a few seconds will hurt your eyes. And if you look long enough, yes, you can go blind.

Eclipses, then, are just as dangerous to look at because, in effect, you are looking directly into the sun. Again, if the eclipse is total, then you're not seeing the sun anymore so it won't hurt you. However, it's difficult to tell when an eclipse is completely total. Even looking at just the outer edge of the sun can damage your eyes. This is also why it's really not a good idea to use binoculars or telescopes or cameras to look at the sun or at an eclipse. All of these focus the light into your eyes even more. And simple filters usually aren't much help.

Listen to the old wives on this one. Looking at an eclipse will more than likely harm your eyes. Will a simple glance make you completely blind? Probably not, but it could damage your eyes, so why chance it? Better to get out that old cardboard box from the closet and see if it still doesn't work. And if it doesn't, there's always the National Geographic.

HOT WATER FREEZES MORE QUICKLY THAN COLD WATER

"In skating over thin ice, our safety is in our speed."
RALPH WALDO EMERSON, *ESSAYS* "PRUDENCE"

If you've ever thrown a party and run out of ice, you've probably heard this one.

The party's in full swing and suddenly you're out of ice. In a panic, you collect all the ice cube trays, and as you start to fill them there's always one person who swears that if you fill the trays with hot water they'll freeze more quickly.

This one isn't true. Hot water does not freeze more quickly than cold water. That's the basic fact. Of course, as with most of these tales, the explanation is a bit more complicated than this.

While it's true that hot water doesn't freeze more quickly than cold water, it *is* true that warm water that has previously been boiled *will* freeze more quickly than cold water straight from the tap. This is because boiled water has fewer air bubbles in it. Air bubbles lower the thermal conductivity of water. Thermal conductivity is how easily heat travels through a substance. The more quickly heat passes through a substance, the faster it cools. So, the fewer the bubbles, the quicker the freeze. And since water that has been boiled does have fewer bubbles, it freezes more quickly.

It also may seem that hot water freezes faster because of the way your freezer works. Water freezes at 32 degrees Fahrenheit. But it will freeze more quickly if the temperature is lower. When you put an ice cube tray full of hot water into the freezer, the thermostat may be affected by the heat coming from the water, making the freezer work harder to lower the temperature. Thus, the water may freeze more quickly. This all depends on how hot the water was in the first place. So it's not the warmth of the water in this case, but the temperature inside the freezer. You could argue, therefore, that a tray full of hot water freezes more quickly than a tray full of cold water, but it really doesn't, given a similar ambient temperature for both trays.

So the next time you're throwing a party, the best thing to do is to stock up on ice so you won't have to make more. And if the party is a real success, you can then consult the chapter on hangovers.

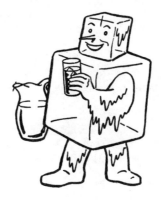

SALTPETER WILL MAKE A MAN IMPOTENT

"Lift not thy hands to It for help—for It
Rolls impotently on as thou or I."
EDWARD FITZ GERALD, *THE RUBÁIYÁT OF OMAR KHAYYÁM*

There's a word in the English language that strikes fear in the hearts of men everywhere. It is a word that turns them from confident studs to paranoid fools. In legend, it has brought more than one man to his knees. This word is . . . "saltpeter."

For those of you not in the know, saltpeter is a simple but legendary mixture that is completely misunderstood. Perhaps it is the word's last two syllables, but somewhere along the way it became associated with limiting a man's ability to perform sexually. Many films over the years have made sniggering references to it, thus adding to its reputation. In fact, it has long been rumored that the army would put saltpeter in soldiers' food to keep their mind on their duty.

The good news for men everywhere is that this is a myth. Saltpeter has nothing to do with putting a damper on one's desire. Instead, it's used as an ingredient in diuretics. Diuretics are used to increase urine output. (For a further, more floral discussion of diuretics, see the chapter on dandelions making you wet the bed.) The chemical name for saltpeter is potassium nitrate.

So if someone sneaks some saltpeter into your food, don't worry about what it will do to you in the bedroom. Better to worry about what will happen to you in the bathroom.

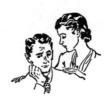

THE TOUCH OF A MENSTRUATING WOMAN
MAKES FOOD SPOIL

....

"God became a man, granted. The devil became a woman."
VICTOR HUGO, *RUY BLAS*

As if women didn't feel lousy enough during menstruation.

There has been much written about menstruation and how
society views it. The fact that it's referred to as "the curse" will
give you an idea how cultures have always looked upon a
woman's period.

There are many old wives' tales that address menstruation.
A few of them are in this book. Others of these include the
belief that if you are menstruating you shouldn't get your teeth
filled at the dentist because the fillings won't stick (not true);
women should not go swimming during their periods (it's up
to them—there's no harm to anyone); women should not exercise when menstruating (also not true); and that there should
be no intercourse during a woman's period (there's no danger in this).

One of the most common superstitions is that a menstruating woman should not handle food of any kind because it will
go bad. The feeling is that when a woman menstruates she is
unclean and/or ill and should avoid touching what others
might eat or drink.

This is an international old wives' tale. In Italy and France,
women are not allowed to make mayonnaise during their time
of the month. In parts of Europe it's believed that women who
touch fruit trees during their periods will ruin the crop. Milk
and wine are also off-limits. French women aren't allowed
near the wineries because of the fear that their "uncleanliness"
will turn the wine to vinegar.

It goes even further than this. Some Italian women will not wash their hair during their periods. You may even have heard of tribes in Africa having menstrual huts, where women live until that monthly problem clears up.

This is all, of course, totally unfounded and not true, nor is this particular old wives' tale true. There is nothing dangerous about a woman touching food when she's menstruating. There's no magical curse that will leap from her finger onto the food or drink. The only possible problem could be that she was so ashamed that she didn't wash herself during her period and was unsanitary because of it. If that were the case then she could pose a hygienic threat, but only because she didn't wash her hands, not because she was having her period.

So this is another tale that is false. Menstruation has nothing to do with food preparation, except, perhaps, that some women would rather not cook if they felt really bad.

CROCODILES CAN GRAB YOUR SHADOW AND PULL YOU INTO THE WATER

"Crocodile rockin' was something shockin' . . ."
ELTON JOHN, "CROCODILE ROCK"

Being city folks, we never really thought about this one too much. There aren't too many crocodiles in the subway, although rumor has it there are some living in the sewers of New York. (Just when you thought it was safe to go back into the bathroom.)

We talked to some people in Florida who live near the Everglades and they said that, yes, this is a common belief and a piece of advice that is passed on to the children and tourists who go near the swamps. And if there's one thing that people want to avoid seeing really close up in that region it's a crocodile.

So what's the truth behind the crocodile tale? Obviously no animal can grab a shadow (even The Shadow knows this). Still, there is some good advice in not getting too close to where a crocodile might be. Many believe that you should stay a certain distance from the water where crocodiles might be lying in wait. The reptiles are very quick and they're also very patient. Usually they'll wait until their victim is very close before attacking. How close is too close? Well, for humans it's considered a good idea to use the length of one's shadow as a guide.

The warning also takes into consideration the crocodile's usual feeding time. How? Well, the animal normally eats around sundown. Fortunately, this is when our shadows are the longest. It's nicely convenient that we stay the farthest away from crocodiles when they are their hungriest.

Believe it or not, this old wives' tale didn't start in the sewers of New York. The Basuto tribe in Africa have long believed that crocodiles have the power to grab onto a man's shadow and pull him into the water. Still, as far as the crocodiles in the sewers are concerned, it's probably a good idea to stay more than the length of your shadow away from an open sewer. If you're closer than that you've got bigger problems than any crocodiles that might be down there.

YOU LOSE MOST OF YOUR BODY HEAT THROUGH YOUR HEAD

"You can leave your hat on."
Joe Cocker, "You Can Leave Your Hat On"

Old wives have always feared cold weather. They think it causes colds (it doesn't) and so whenever anyone is about to go out on a winter's day they insist on bundling them up from their snow boots to their ski cap. Most important, they say, is to be sure to have a hat on when you go outside. They tell you that this is because you lose most of your body heat through your head.

Is this true, or can we tell the old wives to put a lid on it? The answer lies somewhere in-between.

Heat is radiated throughout the human body. The amount and where the heat emanates from depends on what a person is doing at any given time. We can lose anywhere from 7 to 55 percent of total body heat through our heads. The amount depends on how strenuously we're working. If we're exercising, then the heart works harder and faster. This means that more blood is circulated to the head. This, in turn, means that more heat is radiated from the head.

So if you were to exercise on a cold day and not wear a hat, then yes, you would lose a lot of body warmth through your head. Will this make you sick? Not necessarily. It would certainly make you colder, but colds and flu are caused by viruses, not by a change in temperature. So while wearing a hat might make you feel warmer and more comfortable, it isn't a guarantee against catching cold (nor is not wearing a hat an invitation to illness).

The old wives were right about this one. Our hats off to them.

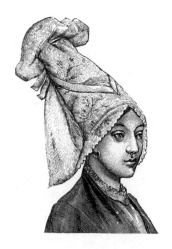

AFTERWORD

est assured that while the complexities of life are never easy to understand, a bit of wisdom from the old wives can always add a touch of laughter and a smile. Part truth, part mysticism, part blind faith, and a dash of good-natured humor, the tales spun by these sages will be with us forever. Of course, as you have seen, they are not always correct. But then, who is? Indeed, while we have endeavored to give the latest information about every tale we have told, today's truth has a way of being superseded by tomorrow's better truth. Thus, some of our old wives' tales—incorrect today—may find vindication in new science to come.

While there are few guarantees in life, one guarantee you can be sure of is that as our society evolves intellectually and physically, more tales will evolve, too. When they do, look for us to be there to fill you in on the latest unfolding in the weird science of old wives' "talemology."

In the meantime, take a big dose of vitamin C, stop cracking your knuckles, and watch out for crocodiles.

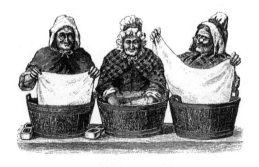